THE OWNER'S GUIDE TO A PRODUCTIVE DENTAL PRACTICE

7 PILLARS EVERY DENTIST NEEDS TO GROW IN THE NEW ECONOMY

TYLER WILLIAMS, D.D.S.

Copyright 2020, Pinecrest Practice Growth LLC.

Any reproduction or use of this book in part or in its entirety, as well as the additional resources is strictly prohibited and will be enforced by law. Author not liable for any action taken by implementing systems and tools discussed in this book.

What Other Practice Owners Have To Say About This Book

"It made me think about my practice and practice growth in new ways. I found your book to be inspiring and encouraging...I think all the 7 pillars can help me - also M.A.P.S.S. to increase my case acceptance."

- Dr. France Nielsen, The Tooth Family Dental, Las Vegas, NV

"Loving your book! So much good stuff I'm reading it slowly...I am excited to take Dr. Williams lead in this, and start implementing some of the concepts presented...I'm going to make it a point to re-read this book again and put a plan to action list in place!"

-Dr. Kevin Van, Captivating Dental Care Clewiston, FL

"I like the idea of constructing your RMAP and looking at what is currently in your practice to help formulate your plan instead of always looking elsewhere...I really enjoyed the information on marketing. To me this is one of the hardest things to navigate, especially as a new dentist. Guidance in this area is priceless and can be a game changer for practice growth."

- Dr. Paul Porter, Avenues Family Dentistry, Salt Lake City, UT

"Your book is applicable to practices of all sizes."

- Dr. Rudy Wolf, Miller & Wolf Family Dentistry, Altavista, Virginia

Unlock Your Free Bonuses,

Videos And Tools For This Book At

yourpracticegrowthbonuses.com

This book is dedicated to you, the private practice owner, and the unique, constantly changing challenges you face each day. I hope that you can learn what has worked for me, thereby saving you time, frustration and energy which you can redirect toward providing the best experience possible for each one of your patients.

Special thanks goes out to my wife and children for their support. I would also like to thank my mentors and colleagues who have helped me achieve the level of success I have reached. I would like to thank my fantastic team at Pinecrest Dental for caring for each one of our patients, for implementing the systems discussed in this book, and for supporting the doctors and practice owners who we aim to help.

Table of Contents

What if Everything You Were Taught About Growing Your Dental Practice Was Wrong? 1

Why Simple Economics is Key to Your Growth 11

How You Need To Practice Differently To Survive Today! 12

Why Better Dentistry Won't Fix Your Practice's Problems 18

What Do You Really Need to Offer Your Patients? 29

Are You Building the 7 Pillars Of a Successful Practice? 36

Pillar #1: Why Marketing Is Your Most Important Practice Tool Today 37

Pillar #2: Why Case Acceptance Is The True Roadblock of Your Practice Growth 52

Pillar #3: What Is The #1 Asset In Your Practice? It's Your People! 72

Pillar #4: Are You Productive or Just Busy? 102

Pillar #5: Creating An Office That Works for You 114

Pillar #6: Ouch! My Billing and Patient Accounts are Out of Control! 122

Pillar #7: What Really Counts at the End of the Day 139

References 155

About Tyler Williams, D.D.S. 157

What if Everything You Were Taught About Growing Your Dental Practice Was Wrong?

- Chapter One -

When I graduated from dental school in 2010 I was beginning my career right in the middle of the Great Recession. Most dentists and small business owners I talked with were constantly complaining about the economy and how "bad" things were in their practices. Two years later I attended a dental research seminar in Seattle, and most of the lunchtime talk was still centered on how insurance companies were robbing us as practice owners and how tough the economy was.

Whether nievely or not, I did not know any differently. I simply kept pressing forward, having nothing but concentrated effort and a positive outlook. I witnessed a dramatic increase in the revenue in my practice each year, and began an existing run with a personal track record of 500 percent growth over the first decade of my career. I don't share this with you to boast, because I've certainly made more mistakes than wins along the way, but I've learned to amplify the magnitude of the wins so that they dramatically overshadow the losses.

I learned a lot about dentistry along the way, and I'm sure you have as well. The problem with most of what we learn about running a dental practice is that it's based on emotions, not on facts.

That didn't work for me.

Staff members hate to do that.

She or he won't want to do that.

Patients only want to do what insurance covers.

Patients only want the cheapest option.

These emotional assumptions are NOT ALWAYS TRUE! While they can be true in certain cases, most practice owners do not have the facts to support these assumptions. I've proven these erroneous thoughts to be wrong time and time again. You were taught in dental school to back up research and studies with facts and data. Shouldn't you be growing your practice following a similar model?

I won't bore you with huge, long studies and pages of charts and graphs. But I will provide you with the key elements you need to take your practice to the next level. By implementing the teachings in this book, I hope, and believe, that you can double your practice in the next 12 months if you set that goal. You could even double it again the next year if you just open your mind to what the future could hold for you.

The purpose of this book is to share with you what I've learned along the way, and how you can dramatically grow your practice in a shorter amount of time than I did. I learned some things the hard way, on my own. On the other hand, I have been incredibly fortunate to have had some great mentors and advisors along the way. I've spent a lot of time reading and shadowing successful people who were doing and producing more than I had. I also received some bad advice from a handful of poor advisors along the way, from whom I also learned, but in different ways.

My advice to you is, don't try to be a do-it-yourself doctor. Don't try to go it alone. Learn from others who've been there, have skinned their knees, and have overcome challenges. Only take advice from people who are successful financially and are leaders. Avoid advice from people who struggle or are broke, as this advice can pull you down to where they are. Instead, be an example of someone who can lift others up by leading the way and by following those who already do.

Don't just read the journals, either. Don't get me wrong--I believe it's important to read the dental journals and magazines several times a year to stay up-to-date on new products and controversial subjects in dentistry. But you should also attend events and success seminars where you can be with like-minded peers who have the right mindset. This will give you a huge advantage over your competitors, most of whom have the wrong mindset. Without the right mindset, it really doesn't matter what you do, you'll struggle.

You absolutely must be part of business, mentoring and mastermind groups outside of your practice, interacting with people who will coach you and push you to reach higher. You can only get so far on your own and, just as I did, you may start to plateau if you aren't constantly innovating and leading your team. If you aren't up for this challenge, I invite you to stop here for a moment and write down what you love about your practice and what you hate about it. If your hate column outweighs the love column, you need to make some major changes in what you do, find a partner, or possibly sell your practice to someone else who likes to do what you hate to do.

If your love column is your clear winner, then you should congratulate yourself on the progress you've made already. Then go to work on finding ways to free up, delegate or change the things you hate so that someone who loves them can take over or outsource them so you can free up your time to focus on the things you love to do. Do not simply work in your practice--turn your practice into a well-oiled machine that works for you. If you'd like some help and ideas in these areas, this book is just for you.

There are two incredibly important things I have learned, and would like to share with you. You'll need these to be an ultra-successful practice owner and to meet your life goals:

1. Construct an RMAP--Relationship Marketing Action Plan--using the tools and 7 Pillars we'll discuss later in this book.

2. Find how to make the plan work FOR YOU and your practice and patients by recruiting, training and retaining the kind of people who are a good match for your practice vision.

Simply trying to grab ideas from various journals, magazines and Facebook groups is not a plan. These are merely ideas and tactics. The same goes for letting sales people at the booths of your local dental convention tell you how to run your practice. They are not practice owners and have not been in your shoes. Should you leverage their advice? Yes. Are most of them good people? Absolutely. But your #1 job as a practice owner is to be the fearless leader who spends time working on the practice as well as being a compassionate provider in the practice.

Unfortunately, most of us are taught this way in dental school. We can barely fit clinical comprehension into four years, let alone practice management, human resources and marketing. This is why you are here--because you want to do more and build an independent practice that suits your lifestyle.

The better method is create your practice vision in this way:

A. Make a PLAN (your "RMAP").

B. Devise STRATEGIES that meet your plan's objectives.

C. Use TACTICS that will push you toward your goals every day.

Create your vision in that exact order. If I were going to build a house, I wouldn't show up to the hardware store and start buying random tools, wood and parts. In the same way, you wouldn't do this for your patients who are in need of a comprehensive treatment plan. You have to be the architect of your practice RMAP marketing plan first, employ the 7 Pillars of strategy next, and then implement your techniques and tactics last.

On the flipside, you shouldn't listen too much to any one consultant or advisor. Nor should you take advice from someone else's perspective and then do the opposite in order to make the right decision. Don't ignore the details or real facts: burying your head in the sand doesn't pay off. Pursuing a degree in economics taught me to always consider the other's perspective in order to truly understand it. To paraphrase a hero of mine, marketing legend Dan Kennedy, you can't say somebody is wrong unless you have read their book and really know who they are and what they are about. Kennedy was not a fan of President Obama, but argued that you couldn't say he wasn't a good president, or criticize him at the dinner table, unless you had read his books first. There is a lot of sound advice in that statement. Take the time to understand who people really are.

There's an old story told by Roger Cromwell, the first president and founder of Temple University, who was also a well-known Baptist minister, lawyer, and writer. He tells of a priest offering advice to a man named Ali, looking for diamonds, as written here from his famous speech *Acres of Diamonds* (quoted from AmericanRhetoric.com):

Ali: "Will you tell me where I find diamonds?"

Priest: "Diamonds! What do you want with diamonds?"

Ali: "Why, I wish to be immensely rich."

Priest: "Well, then, go along and find them. That is all you have to do; go and find them, and then you have them."

Ali: "But I don't know where to go."

Priest: "Well, if you will find a river that runs through white sands, between high mountains, in those white sands you will always find diamonds."

Ali: "I don't believe there is any such river."

Priest: "Oh yes, there are plenty of them. All you have to do is to go and find them, and then you have them."

Ali sold his farm, traveled the world, became impoverished, and eventually lost his life, without finding his treasure. The man who later bought Ali's farm was down by the river one day on the farm property, where his camel was drinking. The man saw a shimmering light in the river and found a large deposit of diamonds, making him rich above his wildest dreams.

Often the "diamonds" in your practice are right under your nose. We can become tempted to look for new shiny objects in the form of new patients and new procedures, but can easily neglect what is right under our noses.

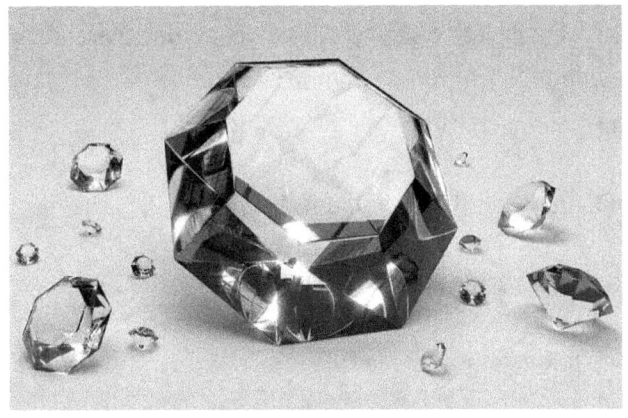

Image source: pixabay.com

DON'T NEGLECT your #1 asset in your practice - your patient list. It is far more valuable than any 3D technology or your entire building. Your patient list IS the goose that lays the golden eggs, so don't neglect it. Nourish it, dig deep, cultivate your list and maximize the value that is already under your feet. This includes your team members. Take care of those around you, not just in the form of dental treatment, but in building long-lasting relationships using the 5R relationship marketing system.

Kennedy (whom I referred to above) has a powerful saying, which goes:

"You don't get a customer to make a sale,

you make a sale to get a customer."

Kennedy is very thoughtful when it comes to his "herd," answering letters and faxes he receives with a personal response-- sending an old-fashioned letter in an envelope. Kennedy doesn't use email, finding it too distracting, unproductive and impersonal. I agree with him in many ways. I have adapted his saying for my practice. You, too, should implement this concept into your office culture as well if you really want to stand out from the crowd and make your RMAP work for you. My practice growth version of his quote is:

"You don't get a patient to do treatment on,

you offer treatment to gain trust with a new patient."

Finding and keeping great patients is THE hardest thing you will do in your practice. This is more difficult than any surgical, restorative or orthodontic procedure you offer--by a long shot. I would take doing a difficult treatment on a great patient over a simple procedure on a difficult patient any day. You probably would, too. How do I define a "difficult" patient? Simply put, a difficult patient is one who is not a good match for your practice. Doing the right thing goes far beyond creating a winning smile for your patients-- it also means being a resource for people who are not a good fit for your practice, so that they can get the help they need. Sometimes this means you'll refer them somewhere else-- but make sure you do it the right way, with a spirit of sincere service and compassion.

If you gain nothing else from this book, please nail down this concept. Not only will it make your job easier and your marketing way more effective, but it will easily make you <u>tens of thousands of dollars, or even hundreds of thousands of dollars per year!</u>

In this book, I'll share with you what I've discovered over the past decade in growing my practice and the kind of patients and team members with whom I love working. I'll share how I have grown my practice by more than 500 percent by creating marketing systems that build and strengthen patient relationships. I will also show you how to recruit the right kind of team members that will help you build your vision into the type of growing practice you've always wanted--one that will support your personal mission statement and life goals.

In Part 1, you'll learn about the Simple Economics of Dentistry Today, including the reasons why simply being a better dentist or taking more CE courses is not the answer to growing your practice. Although offering the best, most comprehensive and ethical dentistry is important, in today's economy, that is not a bonus to your patients--it's expected! Being a great dentist is just your starting point. You'll learn why you are up against a huge wall, and how to get around it.

In Part 2, you'll discover the 7 Pillars to a successful practice, how you can apply them to dramatically enhance the growth curve of your business, and how to create a long-term asset that works **for you**--not just one in which you work. Highlight this book, dog-ear the pages, write notes in it, and most importantly, take action today. Share some of these ideas with your key team members, and make a difference in the lives of your patients, your team members and your family. Now, roll your sleeves up and let's jump in!

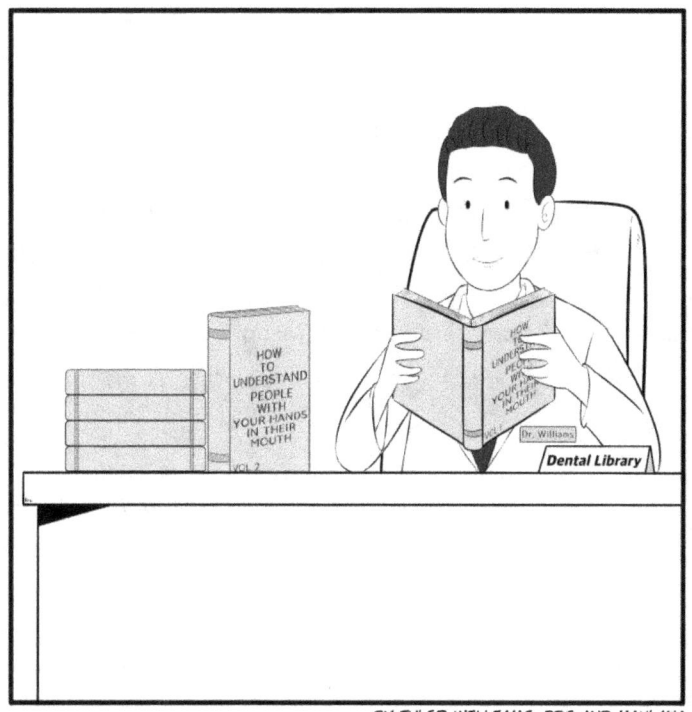

BY TYLER WILLIAMS, DDS AND MAULANA

Chapter 1 Summary:

- Think long term relationships, not just a "quick buck" in providing treatment and growing your patient base.

- Use the Patient Relationship Marketing Rule: You don't get a new patient to do treatment on, you offer treatment to gain trust with a new patient."

- Patients put off dental care when they don't see personalized value in it, and when they don't feel your recommendations meet their needs and desires.

- Create a win-win-win practice that benefits your team, your patients, and you!

Part -1

WHY SIMPLE ECONOMICS IS KEY TO YOUR GROWTH

How You Need To Practice Differently To Survive Today!

- Chapter Two -

Why did you become a dentist? This chapter will help you to rethink your priorities and what you are actually doing for your patients. Focusing on teeth is important, but it's also important to zoom out and take a look through the lens of your patients and their families to gain their perspective.

Why do they choose to come to you?

What are they looking for in a dentist or healthcare provider?

What do they expect from you, and how is the dental workforce changing around you?

The landscape of dentistry is changing. Downward pressures from insurance companies, DSOs, and corporate dentistry are closing in around you, and increasing the costs to run a business. Walmart is now a major player in dentistry and healthcare as well, with CVS not far behind. (If you position yourself properly, however, these high-volume, low-experience clinics shouldn't be a true threat to you. If you'd like to strategize more about this, I'll share my contact info later in this book along with some FREE bonuses for you.)

What's the #1 reason patients put off or don't accept your treatment recommendations? **It's not price. It's not your skills. It's not insurance.** (These are all fables that I was taught when I was first getting into practice that have been proven wrong time and time again.) It's because **they don't see the real need and real value of getting their dental treatment done <u>now</u>**.

People HATE going to the dentist. I always knew there had to be a way to make people feel better about their dental visits. When you look at the top reasons people avoid coming to see you, they include these three common concerns:

1. Lack of perceived need -- they see no real urgency in receiving dental care right now.
2. Fear of the treatment you offer as a dentist.
3. Not enough value --they are unwilling or unable to spend money on your services.

One reason I got into practice ownership was because I was on a mission to change this negative perception of our profession. I was unwilling to definitively accept that people had to dread coming in to have their teeth cleaned or to have work done. I learned this in my heavily subsidized dental school, where we still had sky-high no-show rates in the clinic, even though costs to patients were minimal. Sure, there are other socio-economic reasons why people didn't come to our low-cost clinic, but seeing the value in their own health and in themselves was a huge factor.

In dental school, your patients could receive a crown, filling, or cleaning for a fraction of the cost in private practice. I bet you had some high no-shows at certain times, too. Taking the practical boards exam probably caused nervous panics in many of your classmates. It was a crazy time, but a valuable learning experience.

Within a few weeks of graduating dental school, I was working several days a week in a couple of multi-office, multi-doctor type private practices. One practice was a Medicaid, "take every insurance plan known to man" type of office; and the other was a nicer, but still insurance-driven, practice. I cannot say enough about how much I learned in these offices while I was shopping around, doing research on buying my own practice. I learned what I liked about what these other practices were doing, as well as what I DID NOT like about the way they practiced. I'm not talking about the actual treatment or the ethics of the office--that was fine. What I didn't like was how they attracted patients, herding people in just to squeeze their benefits. It is a working model that is commonplace today, but it wasn't for me. This was not representative of the type of people with whom I wanted to build a working life.

So, I set out to design a practice model that was a win-win-win for my patients, my team and me. Within six months of graduation, late in 2010, I purchased a practice from a retiring dentist in a walk-away sale transaction. He was out and I was in on the same day. I was flying solo, with some mentoring from him, but also relying on the notes, experience and ideas I'd brought with me from dental school, and my few months working in private practice.

Boy, was I about to get hit with the wild storm of reality!

Which insurance plans should I accept, if any? How should I attract new patients? What hours and days should we be open? How do I handle family? Treatment options? Getting in touch with his existing patients? Should I market to new patients? What equipment should I upgrade or invest in? What payroll company should I use? What legal structure do I need? Should I use digital X-ray and practice management software?

It was an older, but clean and well organized office. I inherited his one employee, a dental assistant, who also worked the front desk. Each room had different paint, decor and/or wallpaper, as well as a corded phone mounted to each wall. My predecessor was a very caring dentist who truly went the extra mile for his patients. He offered them all kinds of advice--not just about their oral health, but also about life, retirement planning, raising kids, etc. He was a very intellectual doctor and had shared the office with a partner for years, in an old fashioned, split-expenses type of practice, before his partner passed away. It worked well for him and for the patient demand existing at that time throughout the '70s, '80s and '90s.

Three years later, when I saw the writing on the wall for the old building I was practicing in, I purchased another similar, one-doctor, one-employee practice. I moved my existing small practice over to this new practice. But the recession had hit my new landlord hard, and maintenance had been deferred in many areas of the building, with multiple vacancies existing. I realized that I needed to get out before they bulldozed the building or sold it off to someone else. So, I found another retiring dentist and purchased his practice, (this time a bit wiser and more keen to the numbers, thanks to my undergraduate training in economics), and merged the two practices together. In the meantime, we did a light remodel on the new location and moved everything in three months later.

I was just getting my toes wet in real, private practice dentistry. I could never have predicted my experiences in getting into private practice, both as an associate and an owner, at that time in life. I spent many hours lying in bed at night, pondering my decisions, and making my wife nervous about the additional debt and liabilities I took on as a practice owner. I am forever grateful for my experiences and the mentoring I received. It all helped me to develop relationships with the many great patients we inherited, as I began to truly care for them. What I didn't realize at the time was that my experiences were providing me with real market research about my patients and telling me what I really should be focusing my attention on.

Seek solid advice

I sought advice from many different dentists, professionals, advisors and sales people as I planned, bought and grew my practice. I am forever grateful for the sound and proven advice I received over the years. I can never repay those who have shared with me their motivating, inspiring and proven principles and ideas, all of which have helped me grow personally and professionally. But I also received lots of "bad" advice from people who had mixed agendas, lack of supporting data, or proven results to share. Even surveying your own patients can do a lot more in helping you build your future than some "advice" or "blog post" that lacks a solid foundation. Warren Buffett was quoted as saying, "Wall Street is the only place that people ride to in a Rolls Royce to get advice from those who take the subway." More people lose money trying to make it big in stocks than those who have been truly successful. Don't take advice from someone without experience. You must be the captain of your own shop.

You have your own story about how you got to where you are today. Whether you are in private practice, own a practice, or work at several offices, you can grow your practice, income and patient relationships with the 7 Pillars discussed in this book. You will be able to put together your complete "RMAP" - Relationship Marketing Action Plan to change your practice forever and work with the people for whom you can provide the best care.

Now that we've covered why your patients may avoid stepping in your door, as well as what you need to know to prepare for growth and the RMAP you need to create, we'll move into the demand your patients are creating compared to the supply we are outputting from dental schools.

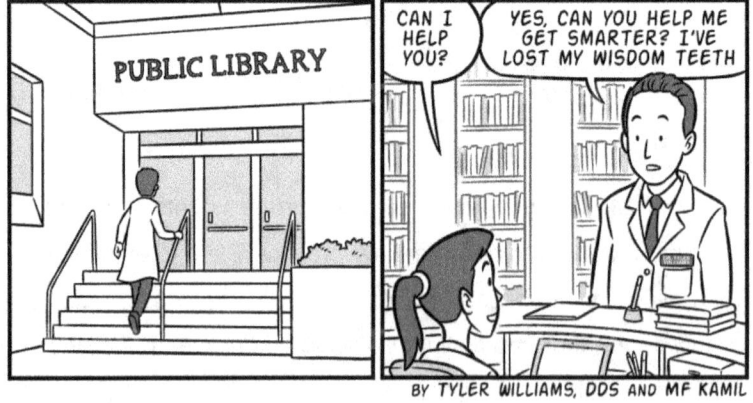

BY TYLER WILLIAMS, DDS AND MF KAMIL

Chapter 2 Summary:

- *When a patient declines treatment, they have just a few choices: put off care until later down the road, do nothing, find an alternative (such as direct aligners or store bought whitening), or switch dentists.*

- *Common reasons your patients choose not to have dental work done in your office include: lack of perceived need, not offering multiple payment options, as well as fear and anxiety about treatment.*

- *The #1 reason your patients say "no" to your treatment plans is when you are not offering enough value in your recommendations.*

- *Always be honest and direct, but making treatment sound too complicated significantly drops your case acceptance rate.*

- *Make sure you take financial and practice growth advice from professionals, advisors and experts who are trustworthy and have real world experience in both marketing and the dental industry.*

Why Better Dentistry Won't Fix Your Practice's Problems

- Chapter Three -

In this chapter, we will discuss today's oversupply of dentists, which unfortunately isn't making things any easier for you. Nearly every community in the U.S. (with the exception of some rural areas) has enough or more than enough dentists to meet its basic needs. You must have a different approach. Don't swim in the waters that are already saturated. Go to the other side of the pond to meet the (often unspoken) needs and wants of your patients who really want to have a winning smile. You'll learn how to navigate these waters so that you can make decisions based on real numbers, not emotions. You'll need facts and faith, but leave the emotions behind if you want to be a leadership-oriented practice owner.

You probably went into dentistry because you are a good person who wants to help people. You likely enjoyed the life sciences or clinical dentistry and decided that you wanted to make it a career. Most dentists I know get into this business for the right reasons. In my graduating class of approximately 100 dental students, there were maybe only two or three whom I wouldn't trust to care for my own family members. The majority of them were dedicated, ethical, and skilled dentists in the making.

When you graduate dental school, you are really just getting started with your education. Your experience in professional school was just the beginning, not the end. Many college graduates see getting a degree as 80 percent of the work and then finding a job and working for life as the remaining 20 percent of the work. I see it as the opposite. When you become a doctor, you have taken an oath to "do no harm" and to treat your patients like you would your spouse or parent. The trouble today is that most people do not plan to constantly challenge and push themselves to be better at their profession, and, most importantly, to continue to provide more value in the marketplace.

Supply what the market isn't demanding at your own peril

Don't fall into the trap of thinking that by holding a degree, you are somehow entitled to a certain income or stream of new patients. This is very shortsighted. This type of thinking may serve you for a short time, but unless you are continually investing your time and money into what your patients and prospects are looking for, I do not believe you truly have your patients' best interests in mind. Graduating from dental or medical school is just the beginning of your learning on how to deliver real value for your marketplace of patients, not the end of it.

You are pushing a huge boulder uphill if you simply believe that a greater "supply" of dental care will make your lives better, your team happier, or bring you more chairside production. I'm here to tell you that I once thought that way, too. But then, however, I reviewed my training in supply and demand through my previous economics background and implemented those ideas. Finally, I saw the big picture. Then I applied these principles to growing my dental practice, and I have since found great satisfaction in helping practices just like yours implement them and succeed.

Just doing more dentistry or taking a few CE courses every year doesn't cut it anymore!

According to a Feb 2020 report by Becker's Dental:

> *At its new clinic in Calhoun, Ga., Walmart Health is offering consumers $30 medical checkups and $25 teeth cleanings, according to*

> Bloomberg...The 12-room, 6,500-square-foot center is designed to compete with CVS and Amazon. Along with an in-house pharmacy, the clinic offers patients diagnostic labs tests, X-rays, eye care and other dental services...However, it's unclear how consumers will respond to the clinic. A survey by CivicScience in September 2019 showed 11 percent of Americans polled would "likely" visit a Walmart Clinic. Walmart Health has also not released information on the number of clinics it plans to open. Along with competing for consumers, Walmart Health may find it hard to recruit dentists and other clinicians, reports Bloomberg. One clinician thought Walmart's listing for a position at the health center was a spam posting.

You may be alarmed at the incredibly low, undercutting fees Walmart is offering here. This will cause a shakeup for nearby practices. My practice is located just a few miles away from Walmart, and while they don't have a dental clinic yet, it's only a matter of time. However, I am not that concerned about it at this point. It will probably fill a great need. If Walmart is selling apples, you need to sell oranges. Be different. The real telling truth here is that ONLY 11 percent of those surveyed said they were likely to visit a Walmart for dental services. The real issue in getting more people to the dentist is contained within understanding why 50 percent or more of your community has not seen a dentist in the past 12 months. These are not all unemployed and financially unable prospects, either. They are doctors, accountants, stay-at-home moms and blue collar workers. They are real people with real needs. How do you reach them? How do you build stronger relationships with your existing patients, so that they will come see you more often?

Supply vs demand

The answer is in the DEMAND of our consumers, _not_ in what you want to SUPPLY to them. Your patients like you, but they don't truly care about how good you are at prepping a crown. They care about how much you care about THEM, and what THEIR best options are.

Just how many dentists does our country actually NEED? In a 2015 JADA article, *Rethinking Dentist Shortages,* the findings concluded that, "there is strong evidence of significant unused capacity within the dental care system today." More than one out of three dentists have reported that they are "not busy enough," according to the study. That means one-third or more of us could go away, and we'd still have enough dentists based on our current levels of production.

> "...Busyness levels have been decreasing, open chair time has been increasing, and appointment waiting times have decreased in recent years. As the supply of dentists in the market increases in the coming years, and given the stagnant aggregate demand for dental care, busyness levels could continue to decrease. However, the data are crystal clear: the dental care system today, in aggregate, has significant unused capacity.
>
> The fact that there is significant unused capacity within the dental care system and that the most important barriers to dental care are financial leads to an important policy implication. In the current situation, adding additional dental care providers to the market is unlikely to address the most critical issues concerning access to dental care. Rather, the evidence strongly suggests that policy makers ought to focus on solutions that address the demand-side constraints the US population faces..."

Current workforce trends

According to a 2019 ADA report, "as of 2019, there are 200,419 dentists working in dentistry (dentists using their dental degree in some fashion) in the U.S." The national average as of 2019 was 61 dentists per 100,000 population. This includes both general dentists and specialists. That means there are about 1,640 patients per dentist in the U.S. today, more or less, by state and area. I don't know about your practice, but if you really want to grow, 1,640 patients may not be enough to hit your goals. Consider that not all of the 1,640 are active patients, either. Other reports have shown that about 40 to 50 percent of the population has not seen a dentist in the past 12 months. In my office, we use 12 months as a guideline of active vs inactive patients. We know many will return after 12 months, but these patients aren't helping your practice grow while they aren't there, for two reasons:

1. These inactive patients are not receiving needed treatment to keep their mouths healthy.
2. These inactive patients aren't boosting your collections.

This is what we call a lose-lose, not a win-win, scenario. But you **can** do things differently and better. You can reach out to those people who have never come into your practice, as well as to those who haven't been in for some time. This book will share some proven methods to help you build your RMAP and get there.

Now, let's develop these numbers a bit further. (I'm a math geek about this stuff, but please, just bear with me, and you'll see how this will help you to make sound business decisions):

> Average number of patients available to you in a given practice area = 1,640.
>
> Average percentage of patients who see the dentist regularly = 50 percent.
>
> Average number of active patients available to you = 820 (1,640 x .5).
>
> Assume that each patient spends, on average, $900 per year (national average).

What could be the average collections per year in your practice?

$900 x 820 = $738,000 average collections per year in your practice.

According to the Health Policy Institute at the ADA, the average general practice collected $717,350 in 2018, and the average specialty practice collected $1,016,080. These numbers are right in line with what our math demonstrates above. You'll have to work a lot harder to gain access to this shared pool of patients, unless you use the 5Rs of the RMAP (Relationship Marketing Action Plan) that we'll describe shortly.

Oversupply of dentists today and in the near future

In 2040, the U.S. population is projected to be 380,000,000. So, assuming that 42 percent of the population (based upon ADA statistics) receives dental care annually, 160 million Americans would have at least one dental visit per year.

If current trends continue, with no further growth in the number of dental school graduates, based on ADA estimates, there will be about 240,000 dentists in 2040. "Estimates assume that about 70 percent (168,000 dentists) would be in full-time practice," the ADA notes.

This suggests that the excess supply of dentists would be between 32 and 110 percent. The study further related that, "at the extreme, even if every person in the United States were to visit a dentist each year, the dentist surplus would be over 25 percent."

According to 2017 research by the Journal of Dental Education about the increasing number of graduating dentists, "whether there will be a painful market-based solution to the problem, as there was in the 1980s, or whether a more orderly path can be found is one of the key challenges of the project." -- from *Advancing Dental Education in the 21st Century*.

Only time will tell us what will occur. The disadvantage you have as a dentist is that you are so highly trained in a specialized area that you may not be useful, nor want another career, if the market becomes way too saturated. You joined the ranks of dentistry because you love helping people and the art and science of working in the mouth. So when everyone else is going to "zig" you need to prepare to "zag." You need to be different in order to grow.

Where you can fall into a trap is by chasing after the WRONG type of patients-- those who ONLY care about insurance, or worse yet, cancel or reschedule 50 percent of the time. Patients who are broke or don't have any credit are also the wrong type of patients to chase. Do these people deserve dental care? Absolutely! Do we all have hard times? Of course. If you have insurance, do you want to use it for medical or dental care? I would. But you can't hold yourself to a false sense of security that these types of patients will help you hit your goals and support your team.

There are resources for patients who can't afford dental care. We have helped to create a charity for low income dental services. Plus, we take in one veteran every year and transform his or her smile on our dime. It is a great honor, privilege, and opportunity to do this. But don't mix business with charity. If you are not the right fit for them, you should help people in need by plugging them into the resources they need to get help. Don't make them search on their own or use "Dr. Google" for help. Be a trusted resource. Have contact info for Medicaid or state run resources on hand so that you can help people in need.

At the same time, there are many patients who are ready to spend far more than the average patient-- many without insurance or knowing that their insurance will not cover their ideal treatment. Go fishing for these patients. It takes more time to build their trust, and they won't come running to you. The best part, however, is that you can spend more time with them and they will appreciate the care you give them much more than the average person would. If you constantly go fishing in the same pond, you'll be tempted to keep signing up for more plans that require you to lower your hard-earned fees or feel that you have to give away more dentistry to compete. I'm here to tell you that's not the case and that's not what I've done to grow my practice.

It's great to work with insurance. If you do accept it, you should be grateful for the collections it can put into your bank account each month. I suggest that you do not become an "insurance-driven" practice, but, instead, opt to become an "insurance-friendly" practice. Always give your patients options based on what they want, not only limited to what insurance covers. Let THEM choose the dentistry that best suits their needs, then support that decision and provide that dentistry to the best of your abilities.

According to the ADA, the American national average is that there are 60.95 dentists per 100,000 people. As of 2019, my state, Utah, ranks 16th in saturation, at 61.05 dentists per 100,000 persons, placing us just about even with the national average. You may wish you could go practice in an area where there are no other dentists and have the entire community at your disposal. But here's the secret--if it's a desirable place to live, there will be other dentists there. Today, there are very few hidden gems that are both great to live in and unknown to the rest of the world.

The right way to create a patient "gold rush"

Don't get caught up in "shiny objects" that are peddled to you. I fell into the snare of spending hours in the convention halls of my local dental meetings when I first got into practice. There were lots of interesting things to see there, but I fell prey to the many sales professionals at the trade booths. I became sold on what they were pitching.

Instead, I've learned to seek out sales professionals who are aligned with my mission and with the tools that I'm looking for to accomplish my goals. If you don't have a plan of action on what exactly you are looking for, then you'll be tossed about by the waves of confusion in the marketplace, and you will keep throwing money into quicksand that won't help to grow your practice on its own.

Be sure to measure every single investment you make. Always ask, "What is my return on this?" ROI (return on investment) is not just measured in the form of money. It's measured in your ROT (return on time), as well as in your health, family, goals, and most importantly, in your relationships, as we'll discuss later in this book. Whatever you are considering buying, implementing or adding to your life, if it's not producing a positive return on your assets, BEWARE!

There is an interesting story about the great Gold Rush of California:

> *On May 12, 1848, a store owner named Sam Brannan held a "one-man parade" to announce the start of the San Francisco Gold Rush.*
>
> *"Gold! Gold from the American River!" Brannan shouted up and down Market Street in San Francisco. He held his hat in one hand and waved a bottle of gold dust in the other. San Franciscans had received false news of gold before. But by all accounts, Brannan's performance sent residents running in search of riches.*

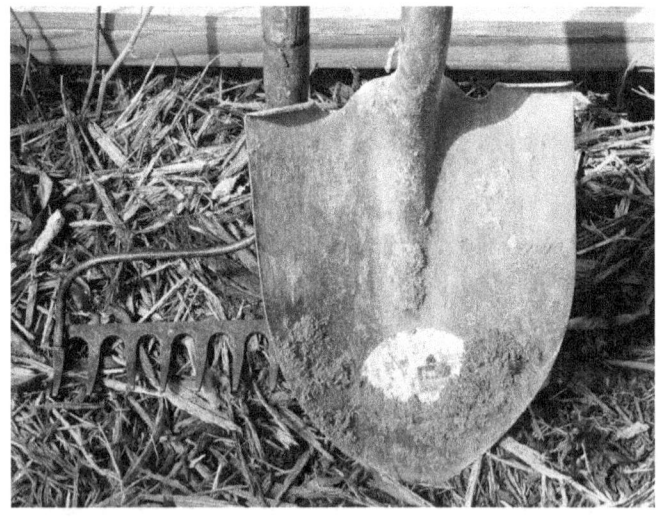

Image Source: pixabay.com

From this period in history came the saying, "during a gold rush, sell shovels." Most of the gold prospectors at this time died broke, lost in the California hills, chasing a pipe dream. Many merchants, traders and general store owners struck it rich providing resources and "shovels" to those who were seeking fortunes. Whether Brannan was honest about the gold or not, I do not know. However, the story provides a valuable lesson - don't get caught up in what is new and shiny. Instead, focus on what people are actually seeking.

Learn the market demand in your area. I cannot tell you what that is, but you must find that niche by doing market research. Whether it's in dentures, implants, cosmetic dentistry, kids' dentistry or sleep apnea, you must find out. You should use a combination of patient surveys, legitimate online research, industry trends, list brokers, and even your local library as resources to find exactly what people are seeking. Your webmaster can provide you with a report on what types of links, keywords and traffic your prospective patients are clicking on in order to find you and other dentists in your area. Don't think you can just supply more gold to your patients--**go to where the demand is**.

In the next chapter we'll cover what you REALLY need to offer your patients to build a growth model that serves you and your team. You'll learn what your patients are actually searching for (maybe even behind your back) and how to anticipate their personal values to better serve them. You'll see the beginnings of your RMAP (Relationship Marketing Action Plan) start to come together as you realize what steps you need to take to build valuable patient relationships that last.

Chapter 3 Summary:

- The dental marketplace is overcrowded as a whole and is only getting more saturated.

- The cost of running a practice is increasing while profit margins in most practices are shrinking.

- The personal incomes of most dentists across the country are stagnant or decreasing.

- Follow this data-driven advice in this book to be different with your practice, or else be caught as one of the "average" at your own peril.

- Rather than just learning more dental procedures, spend your creative energy on finding out what your patients really want.

- Find the consumer demand in your market and build your RMAP upon that.

What Do You Really Need to Offer Your Patients?

- Chapter Four -

In this chapter, you'll learn what and how to offer your patients what they ultimately want. I'll reveal some tips that I use to help my own team members and patients every day and how they can help you maximize your time and energy. Not only will these tips help you to stay on time, but you'll feel confident about the treatment plans you offer, and so will your patients.

As recorded in a recent *Wall Street Journal* online article, in January 1792, "the dollar sign ($) was born and showed up for the very first time on a federal U.S. document, which was a treasury bond issued to President George Washington." This historical event forever changed that universal token of exchange in the way we know the great equalizer of value, money.

Only three stocks have ever broken the trillion dollar mark, but recently, Google's Alphabet stock (GOOG) became the fourth to break the trillion dollar mark. Apple, Amazon and Microsoft are the only others to ever hit this massive valuation. On the flip side, J.P. Morgan Chase, the largest U.S. bank, is worth less than half of Google, Amazon, or Apple,* valuing just short of $426 Billion as of February 2020.

*Full disclosure: I am a previous shareholder of Apple. My iPad was one of my tools for writing this book!!

This brings me to this point: what do your patients really want from you?

All of us NEED a bank account to stay in business or to buy groceries and gas. But most of us only WANT an iPhone, two-day delivery, or online search at our fingertips. These WANTS aren't things we need to function. As a bank holding your money, J.P. Morgan Chase is more of a necessity than any of these tech giants, yet it isn't even worth 50 percent of the value of Google. But do you really NEED Google to have a fulfilling life?

Wants vs needs

When you tell your patients they NEED a crown, mouth guard or wisdom tooth removed, do they believe you? You are clinically trained to know what's best physiologically for your patients, but do you truly understand their psychology?

Helping our patients' WANTS match their needs is the key to case acceptance. If they want whiter teeth, show them how they need a perio treatment to make their teeth whiter. If they want to save their teeth until they die, show them how they need a crown to prevent losing a tooth, a root canal, or dental implant.

As demonstrated by Google, Apple, Amazon and Microsoft, WANTS are at least two times more powerful than needs for all of us.

You may WANT to go and grab an afternoon snack, but surely you don't absolutely need one. Remember, **never underestimate the emotional side of needs from you or your patients.** This powerful psychological principal can **more than double your case acceptance** like it has in my practice.

Have You Studied What Your Captive Market
(Patients In Your Practice) Really Want?

According to the Google Keyword tool, here are some of the top keyword searches for patients researching dentists in 2019:

Keyword	Average # of monthly searches
dentist	1220000
dentist near me	823000
crown	550000
braces	450000
orthodontist	368000
teeth whitening	301000
veneers	301000

In a 2016 study from the *International Journal of Orthodontic Rehabilitation*, factors affecting patients' desire for seeking orthodontic treatment were evaluated. Here's what they found:

Functional need was felt mostly by the males (36%), whereas females felt esthetics to be their major concern (72%). Fifty-three percent of the patients rated their dental appearance as bad and 47% had a teasing experience for protruded teeth. Majority of patients (76%) considered the improvement of general esthetics the most important outcome for seeking orthodontic treatment, whereas 11% sought treatment to improve dental health, 4% to enhance self-confidence, and only 1% to improve chewing and speech.

In my office, we ask patients the following questions about reasons why they are seeking dental treatment. First, when we see a patient for a consultation, we ask the following question:

Which of these factors matter most to your dental health?

1. Appearance of your smile
2. Long lasting dentistry
3. Your comfort
4. Functionality of your teeth

Second, we ask the following question:

When considering treatment options for your care, which of these are concerns for you?

1. Fear of dental work.
2. Lack of trust with dentists.
3. Treatment not important right now.
4. Not the right time for me to have treatment done.
5. Cost of dental care.

The interesting part about this is that many current and future patients will actually cite "treatment not important right now" (aka no real sense of urgency) as a big reason to put off care, but they won't always tell you that unless you dig deep for the answer. The biggest reason we've found that this happens is that we inadvertently confuse them with too much dental jargon or too many options. Remember: a confused mind won't accept treatment.

When you look at different studies, finances are often a factor, but if you drill right down (no pun intended) to the real reasons patients put off or deny treatment, finances are often not the biggest factor. Pain, discomfort, fear, time and wondering if it REALLY needs to be done are bigger factors.

Fear: a (bigger than you think) reason your patients avoid dental care

Whether you know it or not, many of your patients and potential patients avoid receiving your recommended treatment, whether they say it or not, due to fear.

A 2016 Study in PubMed, titled "Dental Fear and Avoidance in Treatment Seekers at a Large, Urban Dental Clinic" reported the following:

> *Over 20% of patients reported elevated anxiety/fear, of which 12.30% reported moderate and 8.75% high fear. Severity of dental anxiety/fear was strongly related to the likelihood of avoiding dental services in the past and related to myriad presenting problems.*

I believe these numbers of fearful patients may be quite a bit higher, depending on where you draw the line for "fearful." I've noticed hundreds of patients over the years start to knuckle up as they grip the armrests, squeezing them tight in preparation of an injection or drilling. One of the best feelings is to hear a patient say, "That was a lot better than I imagined" after you finish their treatment. If you aren't already doing so, you should regularly ask, "Was that worse, about the same, or better than you imagined it would be?" That feedback is priceless!

Today's Baby Boomers grew up in a time when we had belt-driven drills and Novocaine. What a terrible sight to imagine--smoke coming out of your mouth, big needles poking you, and the smell of burning teeth! Why would you want to pay for that torture? Why is dentistry one of the only healthcare professions that insists on drilling and doing surgery without offering at least mild sedation as the standard of care? Of course there are many people who don't need mild sedation, and some who shouldn't have it for medical reasons. You could make a good argument, however, that spending extra time on one longer visit in order to get all of the bacteria and disease out of the mouth is better and healthier for everyone in the long run.

Even with advances in technology, many of your patients don't know how comfortable you can actually make dentistry feel to them. They don't know that you can infiltrate a tooth and avoid a block in many cases. They don't know you can offer them newer buffers and vibration devices to make their injections way more comfortable. Even offering them a pillow, blanket, lip balm or drink of water will go a long way in showing your patients that you really care. They expect great dentistry as the minimum level of care; it's all the extra touches that really set you apart as being different and inspire them to call you "their dentist."

If you don't offer some type of sedation, or at a minimum, nitrous oxide/laughing gas to your patients, I strongly urge you to get whatever licensing, outside professionals, or equipment you need asap to offer this life-changing service to your patients. I've had multiple patients experience some level of dental sedation for the first time, and tell me that, without a doubt, they'll never go back to dental treatment without it. Your case acceptance will go up dramatically by doing this one thing alone.

Now that we've covered the impact on fear in your practice, we'll next discuss why marketing is the number one asset to growing your practice, and how to market in a way that does not come across as sleazy, pushy or as "bad advertising." To recap this chapter, remember that fear not only paralyzes your patients' decisions, it will paralyze yours as well. You can't have a growth mindset if you are living in fear of what the practice next door is doing, or if your patients will leave you because you drop their insurance plan. Remember to ask the right questions and then build them into your treatment plan.

In the next chapter, we'll open up the 7 Pillars, and you'll learn why marketing (which should be relationship-driven in your dental practice) is, and will continue to be, the number one tool to successfully growing your practice in the new economy.

Chapter 4 Summary:

- Use low cost (or even free) market data, online data and postal service data to find out what people are actually searching for and what dental keywords they're looking at in your area.

- Create customized interview questions to ask your patients (both new and existing patients of record) to increase your case acceptance rate.

- Way more patients and prospects are fearful of the dentist than most practice owners and dentists fully appreciate.

- Make your patient experience much more comfortable and you will stand heads and shoulders above the crowd.

Part – 2

ARE YOU BUILDING THE 7 PILLARS OF A SUCCESSFUL PRACTICE?

Pillar #1: Why Marketing Is Your Most Important Practice Tool Today

- Chapter Five -

Now that we've covered fear, you'll learn more about the MOST IMPORTANT Pillar of the 7: Marketing. You may be thinking, "But I'm a dentist. I don't want to market; I want to treat patients!" Yes, you are absolutely right, this is what you want to do most, but you can't treat patients if they don't know who you are and exactly what services you offer. This is where marketing comes in, measured in Return on Investment (ROI).

There are four types of Return on Investment numbers you should measure and monitor in your practice and to achieve a solid growth trajectory:

1. ROT: Return on Time.
2. ROP: Return on People.
3. ROC: Return on Cash.
4. ROM: Return on Marketing.

We'll get more into the details of these later, but for now just simply know that your time is finite on any given day. You can always work more than 40 or 50 hours per week, but it's usually at a diminishing rate of return (ask me how I know - been there, done that). If you measure this in your production or income per hour, it goes down dramatically when you break that amount for a consistent period of time. Sure, you can work extra during those very busy weeks or during your busiest season of the year. But you can't successfully do this for long periods of time.

For example, the week(s) leading up to a vacation, when I will be out of the office for usually two to eight days, I will ask my team to stack the schedule higher and work a bit extra to buffer the production and collections that I know will slacken when I leave. We also plan procedures and doctor coverage accordingly. If you have an associate, this should also factor into your strategy.

Part of your RMAP should be having a plan for caring for your patients who have pain or emergency dentistry needs while you are gone. This is a form of marketing as it is designing a way for your team to articulate this to your patients and how to leverage this to your advantage. In my office we see a bump in same-day treatment before I leave town as people don't want to run a risk of having a problem when I'm gone, so they are more open to having the dentistry done sooner. This is how you get a bump in your ROM (Return on Marketing).

One is a very lonely number

"One is the loneliest number." This famous song by Harry Nilsson topped the Billboard charts in 1969, and its lyrics still ring true today. I remember hearing this song on the oldies station my dad would listen to when I was growing up. If you heard it I'm sure you'd recognize it as well.

Just as the 2020 Coronavirus outbreak began to take hold, *Investor's Business Daily* reported:

> ...Apple warned that it likely will not meet its guidance for the current quarter because of business interruptions related to the outbreak of the current coronavirus strain known as Covid-19...Work is starting to resume around the country, but we are experiencing a slower return to normal conditions than we had anticipated,' the company said in a note to investors. Apple said its worldwide iPhone supply has been constrained by the factory closures in China due to Covid-19.

Then the supply of iPhone parts became even more scarce for Apple as economic conditions worsened. This brings up an important point regarding **your marketing**, and **your source(s) of new patients**.

Marketing is an ugly, sleazy word to many dental practice owners. Many of our colleagues hate the idea of thinking about "advertising" or "sending out postcards" or "putting up office signs." But those things are marketing tactics, not what defines marketing.

Think of marketing as simply a way to get your patients or prospects to ask a question. A great example of this is a classroom of students. Marketing is getting someone to simply raise their hand and express interest. Case acceptance (what other industries call "selling") is getting that student to act on their interest and take the next step.

There are 3 principles to consider when you develop your RMAP - Relationship Marketing Plan:

1. Decide WHO you want to market to.
2. Decide WHAT dental service(s) you want to market.
3. Decide HOW you want to market your services.

The BIGGEST mistake most practice owners make when taking on a marketing project is principle #1 - the WHO you are marketing to. Do you want to see kids, adults, or families? Do you want to treat people who want dentures or implants? Do you want to see people from blue collar neighborhoods or white collar neighborhoods? Study the demographics and psychographics of your area before you buy a practice, send out a postcard or offer a new service. Don't let your marketing "fall on deaf ears" but not know the #1 key to great marketing, the WHO!

Later we'll discuss more about your list - your patients inside of your Practice Management Software and how you can best maximize your relationships with them. But remember, you will be tempted to jump right in to offering a new service or a new marketing tool, without really understanding the area and what people are looking for in your target audience.

A valuable exercise is to look at your current marketing to your sources of new patients and continuous care patients. I could probably guess that Apple has a backup plan in case their sources of electronics in China ever dried up, but can you imagine if your supplier of parts and pieces of your iPhone and other Apple products suddenly cut you off? Can you imagine if your only source of patients was one insurance plan, and that employer moved out of your area or that plan was dropped? You'd *instantly* become an anchor, dead in the water.

What are your best sources of new patients in your practice? How many do you have? Do you review this weekly with your office manager or marketing team?

Today Google changes its algorithm weekly, if not daily. If your new patients come primarily from Google search, like many of ours do, and, out of the blue, Google drops your listing or says your ads are no longer approved, how will this affect your practice?

Imagine you are filling a large bathtub when growthing your practice. Not only do you need to plug the leaks to prevent it draining (and there are always a few leaks that you can never fully stop, but you should contain and slow them to a very small drip), but you also need to constantly find new ways to keep the faucet flowing.

If your practice only has one "faucet" or source for new patients and that faucet breaks, how long until you have it fixed? **In what ways will you be impacted in the meantime?**

Back in 2018, an online "SEO expert" who was managing part of our online marketing allowed Google to change our local listing type into a "hospital/medical practice" instead of a dental office without noticing it, and guess what happened? You got it - boom - instantly, no more new patients from Google for weeks until we figured it out. We weren't coming up on any local searches for the word "dentist" at all. Luckily, since we tracked these numbers on a daily, weekly and monthly basis, we noticed the problem internally and made quick adjustments. We soon had to fire our online listing manager for being so neglectful. His job was to monitor this daily, and he let weeks go by without even noticing - we had to find out about it on our own. The big lesson: never delegate the tracking to anyone else but to your direct team.

Today's "internet marketing gurus" tout all kinds of dashboards and tracking software that is supposed to make this simpler and turnkey for practice owners. Although these can be helpful tools, never let them overshadow your own internal tracking. No one, and I sincerely mean no one, will care about your marketing results like you will. I bet most of your patients are not waiting around for that "new magic software" to send them an alert that you have an opening for a cleaning. Don't forget that most of your patients don't care about dentistry even a tenth as much as you do. They care about their own needs and how you treat them when they call or are in your office.

Fortunately, in the road bump we hit that I related above, this was not our only new patient source, so we recovered just fine and were back up to record production and collection numbers in just a few months. But if we had had no other marketing sources except this one, **we could have been in deep trouble or even financial ruin, especially if we were the size of Apple**. (A big advantage of running a small business is it's usually easier to turn the ship around when you approach dangerous waters like we encountered.) We had more than one "faucet" filling our tub so we weathered the storm and - most importantly - we learned from the experience.

The bottom line message is: always be looking for new ways to improve your current lead sources, and find the new ones that are performing with at least a

3:1 front end ROI. **Make your marketing plan multidimensional, always with a contingency plan.**

Remember, marketing IS NOT advertising. Marketing is sharing your message to a group of people who may be interested in your services. Advertising is simply one of the available arms of marketing that you could use. If you don't like to "advertise" or promote yourself via postcards or email, you have to remember two things:

1. If you choose to not be marketing, that actually IS your form of marketing. Just like many eclectic restaurants and small hipster shops choose to do, word-of-mouth referrals may be your #1 source of marketing. By not going mainstream, or big scale, that is your marketing message and that's okay, as long as it meets your big picture plans and you understand your position.

2. Don't bury your head in the sand. You need to track the results and numbers. As of this writing, Google search, patient/team/doctor referrals and our street sign are our top three sources of producing new patients, and the other ten main forms of marketing we do rotate on a monthly basis on performance.

But this could change at any time. If you practice in a small town or rural area, it can change even faster if one big factory or business moves out of town or outsources their work overseas. You should look at a **3:1 ROI on the front end as the minimum front-end investment** to keep putting your time and money into any given form of marketing. **Anything producing a lower ROI is actually COSTING you time and causing you to LOSE money.**

Here's why.

The average dental practice has 60-80 percent overhead. Let's say you're at 70 percent overhead this year, which includes taxes, payroll (not including you - the owner), operating expenses, rent, etc. With a 30 percent profit margin (after taxes), you need every dollar to produce at least three to one to come out ahead. If you invest $500 in social media marketing to produce $1500 in new patient production, your profit formula is as follows:

> $1500 production x 70% = $1,050 in existing expenses, leaving you with $450 profit. Now subtract your new social media marketing expense of $500 and you end up with -$50 (negative) front end profit. To avoid another $50 loss, you should make an RMAP (Relationship Marketing Action Plan), based on the 5R Relationship Marketing system we teach to utilize one or more of the following three strategies.

1. **Increase your profit margin** to move your profits to a positive number. Examples would be to lower your lab bill, minimize wasted supply budget, evaluate your payroll, etc.

2. **Increase your marketing ROI** to multiply the production. For example, what marketing systems and strategies could move you from 3:1 ROI to 4:1 ROI? This would produce $2000 in new production from a $500 investment, rather than $1500.

3. **Increase your referrals and frequency of patient visits/recare** for increased back end production. You should give any form of new marketing at least three months to see if it gains traction. You can't expect one paid social media post, Google ad or postcard to exponentially multiply overnight. In today's crowded and noisy environment of purchase and marketing everywhere we go, you have to sharpen your skills more than ever, or have someone who has been there help you navigate these turbulent waters.

For example, if your new patient receives $1500 in restorative treatment, and then schedules a hygiene appointment and he refers in and brings in his spouse for treatment, your ROI increases. You paid $500 up front to bring in the right kind of new patient with marketing, plus another $100 for him to bring in his spouse (through newsletters, emails, new patient brochures or packages, referral programs and other retention strategies you use - these aren't free and should be expenses as trackable marketing). Your marketing costs have now increased from $500 to $600. However, he now has $1500 in restorative treatment, $250 in hygiene and his wife receives an additional $950 in treatment. Now your total ROI is 4.5:1, as follows: $2,700 in new production, divided by $600 in marketing investment. By the way, never assume or expect referrals to be "free." Even though you shouldn't be "paying" patients for referrals, there is still a cost to market your programs and services, including labor, materials and promotional materials.

I suggest using a combination of the above, and reevaluating every quarter on how to leverage multiple strategies to improve your profits. Remember, a 3:1 ROI is your bare bones, narrow margin, minimum ROI on any investment in your practice, including team members; 4:1 is good; and 10:1 or higher is your ultimate goal. We have a simple street sign that has produced 33:1 and higher on certain months throughout the year.

Team member efficiency: your biggest and most important investment

One important KPI you should track on your scorecard is team member ROI. We call this "TME," which stands for team member efficiency. Associate doctor compensation and hygienist compensation is more difficult to take above 4:1 ROI on a regular basis due to expectations on pay, but this changes as economic conditions fluctuate. One advantage of an economic downturn is you get more applicants competing for the same position willing to work for lower pay. I'm not suggesting you ever pay someone less than their worth, but rather, measure your compensation by how much value they put into your marketplace-- your team and your patients. We'll discuss more about team member efficiency later in the book in the 'People" chapter.

To make up for this typically minimum acceptable return, utilize your other team members to give this return a boost, and especially utilize your best marketing to take your ROI above 4:1, to bring up the average return on investment.

One of the most common questions I see practice owners ask, is, "How much should I pay my hygienist?" To answer this, you must first reframe the question as, "How much does my hygienist want to make, per year, that is fair to both of us?" There's a huge difference in take-home pay for a hygienist working one or two half days per week, versus a hygienist who works five days a week. The two have completely different circumstances and goals.

Use your calculator - if the math doesn't work, nothing else will

Do the math backwards. Start with how much a hygienist would like to make each day, then multiply this number by four. Now you have your per-day adjusted production goal for the hygienist, including any incentives. Now, future out how you can make this TME number go to 4.5:1, 5:1 or higher. This creates a growth mindset and incentivizes your hygienist. If you want to grow, and your hygienist doesn't, you have just weeded out the problem and have the tools to make necessary adjustments.

For example, calculate what you pay your hygienist per hour, including payroll taxes and benefits. Multiply that by four, and that's what you should average per hour in net production per hygienist. If you are below that number, you need to tighten up your schedule or adjust your fees to a more profitable level. If you are above that number, boost your marketing because you have a goose that is laying golden eggs. Based on a 75 percent average overhead practice, you'll need a 4:1 minimum on hygiene. Here's an example:

- $150 per hour hygiene net production / 4 = $37.5

- In reverse, if you are paying your hygienist $40 per hour (including payroll taxes and benefits (those are a real factor), you may be actually losing money on each hygiene patient at $150/hour production. Hygiene should not be a "loss leader" just to get more doctor production, as some people say.

- Instead, multiply the $40 per hour x 4, which equals $160, and now you have your MINIMUM net production per hour you need to create hygiene. At least $240 per hour would give your practice a 6:1+ ROI.

You should do the same exercise for front office team members and assistants, which can provide an even better ROI depending on your procedure mix. Once you've calculated your marketing and team member ROI, weigh this against other forms of investments you could make, such as the stock market, real estate, etc. Don't join the many dentists who get sucked into traps of unfamiliar business territory, when you could make a better ROI in the practice you already have working for you by simply making your marketing better.

Another quick and valuable way to boost your hygiene "TME" to 4:1 and up, is to take advantage of add-on services such as fluoride varnish and dental sealants. Often adding a few of those in per day can be all the difference to go from a 3:1 to 4:1, or from a 4:1 to a 5:1 and above.

Some examples of increasing case acceptance for these valuable services in your hygiene department include:

- A guarantee (yes I know you cannot usually guarantee results but you have to dig deep to find something you can guarantee to take the risk out of it for your patient - be creative!)

- Social proof - such as why 85 or 95 percent of your patients elect to have this done, etc.

- Stories

- Consultative recommendations (valuable to both your team member and your patient) vs simply making a transaction (where a win - lose relationship exists)

Add-on services that mutually benefit your hygienist and your patients include:

- Bonded sealants
- Same-day whitening
- Varnish
- Gum therapy
- Electric toothbrushes and irrigators

A great rule of thumb is that you should always strive to deliver more value to your patients than that for which they are paying you. You may be guilty of doing it the other way around, or giving away treatment for which you should be charging. You can't go broke being a nice guy or gal, and expect to develop your team and reach your goals.

By incentivizing your team members to make and help your patients stay healthier, everybody wins. In the long run, it saves your patients thousands of dollars as well as pain through avoiding preventable dental care and other interrelated medical issues.

The magic number of ROI

<u>The magic secret of increasing returns is, when your ROI goes up, so does your patient loyalty and the quality of your patient experience.</u>

I'll repeat that for you one more time: when your ROI goes up, so does your patient loyalty and the quality of your patient experience! How could that be? Because the more you produce in your office, the more value you are giving your patients - value in your marketplace. Increasing your ROI forces you to boost your practice value, improve your systems and run a consistent operation for your patients. It forces you and your team to do some big thinking and create a growing, thriving practice.

Try a lot of things and test everything. As direct mail pro Keith Lee says, "Test small, tweak again, get dialed in, and then roll it out. My biggest mistakes were when I looked at some marketing thing and said, this can't fail. And I went out and did a big start without testing it." You wouldn't have prepped a crown for a real patient during your first day of dental school; you had to start small by practicing on a dentoform or model and work your way up until you could prep multiple units or arches at once. Test, remove what doesn't work, and ramp up what does. This is your golden ticket to making your RMAP a success. You'll have to accept that not every strategy you deploy will work out perfectly, but your big winners will be home runs that will more than make up the difference.

Make sure to give your business card/contact information to prospective patients, and update it for existing patients. This is the gold in the gold mine of your dental practice. If the power is cut off in your building, you can't provide any treatment for your patients, but more importantly, if communication is cut off from your patients they won't know what you're offering or how to get in touch with you.

Free vs no-so-free

Often, it is just as difficult to get a potential patient to grasp onto something that you are offering them for free as it is to get them to grasp onto something that costs money. Many of your patients are incredibly fearful of needles or drills or having work done in their mouth. These patients wouldn't even let you pay them to have certain dental procedures done because they are terrified of these procedures. So when you think of marketing, don't think you have to give away a whole bunch of free stuff to do well. In fact, sometimes the opposite is true. Many people are skeptical of "free" options and would rather pay for something they see as valuable.

It is worth your time to test both free offers and paid offers, but be careful not to undercut or de-value the many years of education you've put into becoming a great dentist. The more you look and sound like a commodity, the more the public will perceive dentistry that way. So, at the end of the day, remember that it's not necessarily the cost to the patient or potential patient that you need to think about when marketing. It's the level of value you can add to their life, by giving them a winning smile, or in making them feel more confident. Role-play this with your team and ask them to articulate the value of being a patient at your practice. If they can't put it into words, then you know where your challenges lie, as well as where opportunities lie.

Do multi-method, multi-strategy marketing

The highly successful marketer Jim Rohn promoted the principle of "massive action." This means implementing multiple strategies at once. Think of the human body as a marketing plan: principal (the body), strategies (the arms and legs) and tactics (fingers and toes). As dentists, we tend to want to jump right into tactics. It's amazing how much we love to "talk shop" about dentistry. It's our passion. We focus on the type of bonding agent, implant or ceramic we want to use. That's the science we love; it's what we're interested in and what gets us excited to discuss. But before you can dive right into tactics, you must write down the principals of your marketing plan and the reasons why you do what you do. Just like the well-written book by Simon Sinek says, "*Start With Why.*" Then have your team help you create and implement the strategies and execute the tactics needed to be successful.

If you want to be really successful with restorative, surgical or orthodontic dentistry, you need to have a comprehensive plan. Marketing is the same. Your plan doesn't need to be complicated - I've built both simple and complex marketing systems, and sometimes the simple ones outperform. But your marketing plan does need a marketing calendar and follow-up on a weekly basis to grow your practice. You'll want to market through different methods, such as a patient newsletter, email and your on-hold messaging system (just remember not to keep your new patients or your existing patients trying to schedule on hold - this is a real trust-killer).

Start small, test what works, then add to it, just like you do with your team members and your personal value. Always keep the ROI accountable on your marketing, and remember, most of the rewards in a dental practice are on the back end, not the front end. **To build a successful relationship marketing system (RMAP) you perform dentistry to get a patient, not the other way around.**

The target minimum ROI you should shoot for on all marketing activities (essentially defined as everything your practice does, whether you look at it direct or indirect marketing) is 13 to 1. We calculate this as follows:

Total monthly collections / Total marketing budget = Marketing Total ROI

This is what keeps your patients coming back. Everything from refreshments in your reception area, to Netflix on tablets, to your website and emails you send to patients is factored into your marketing budget. This is what builds your growth-oriented practice.

Before we end this chapter, I strongly advise that you put personality into your marketing. Look for vendors who, through doing what they do best, will help make your life easier; but use your marketing to share your personal story and personal brand. Remember: *people care much more about WHO you are compared to WHAT dental procedures you offer*. People want to do business with people they know and trust.

Bonus: If you don't want to build your RMAP - relationship marketing action plan, there are people who can help you create and implement this. You may visit yourpracticegrowthbonuses.com for extra bonuses and videos, or to contact me to schedule a free 30-minute RMAP assessment of your practice.

Chapter 5 Summary:

- Marketing systems are the #1 most important systems in your practice.

- Learn the four types of practice return on investments (ROI): ROT (return on time), ROP (return on people), ROC (return on cash) and ROM (return on marketing).

- One is the loneliest number; don't become too reliant on any one type of patient attraction or patient retention media type or strategy.

- Decide who you want to market to, what specific services you want to market (and avoid), and how you are going to market them. Then develop your procedure mix.

- Don't be a "Jack of All Trades," or try to be everything to everyone - otherwise you won't be anything to anyone.

- The minimum return on investment you should aim for in order to have a successful ROI is 3:1 on the front end.

- Build your RMAP and execute it monthly (your relationship marketing action plan).

- Team members are your best and most valuable marketing tool.

Pillar #2: Why Case Acceptance Is The True Roadblock of Your Practice Growth

- Chapter Six -

When your patients accept your treatment, it is called "Case Acceptance." Others may call this selling, and you may hate that word, but in dentistry we *are* selling, but in the most ethical, honest and transparent way. Selling is simply closing the deal, and it's the only way you'll ever pay your bills while you grow your practice. In this chapter, you'll learn how to boost your case acceptance--even double it, way above the national average.

You may alternately refer to case acceptance as "retention" of your patients. We use these terms interchangeably because in a general practice, 99 percent of your patients should have a next visit scheduled when they leave. Hygiene, restorative dentistry, elective procedures, or even a suture removal or phone consultation should all be scheduled. Everyone should have their next step discussed and approved by them. It's your ethical and professional obligation to take care of their needs. If you sincerely believe what you do is valuable to your patients, then don't hide it. Get their feelings and questions out on the table and decide together what is most important to them, then tie it to the next step. This is the way you should measure how well you've retained your patient relationships.

We'll get more into the "how" in just a minute, but first I'd like to share with you a story from successful copyrighted entrepreneur "Doberman Dan."

> *A door-to-door vacuum cleaner salesman managed to finagle his way into a woman's home in rural Alabama.*

> *"This machine is the best ever," he exclaims, while pouring a bag of dirt all over the living room floor.*
>
> *The woman expressed her concern that the vacuum cleaner might not be able to clean up all the dirt.*
>
> *So the salesman made what he believed to be an irresistible offer…*
>
> *"If this machine doesn't completely remove all the dust and dirt, I'll lick it off myself."*
>
> *To which the woman replies, "Do you want ketchup on it? We're not connected (to) electricity yet."*

This story is both instructive and unfortunately true. Just as in sales, as dentists we are too quick to offer a treatment or solution that can often fall on "deaf ears," or in other words, is the wrong treatment for *that person.*

People are more informed than ever today, and often have their mind already made up about what they want before they even see you. So make sure you are offering the right treatment to the right person, and if someone isn't ready for it yet, simply nurture the relationship and/or start with a lesser or smaller treatment. As you earn their trust, eventually the seeds you plant will turn into a fruitful tree for both you and your patients.

How do you increase case acceptance?

Famous early 1900s author Robert Collier wrote, "Enter the conversation already going on in your prospect's mind." As mentioned earlier in the supply vs. demand comparison, too often as dentists, we try to convince our patients to get the treatment *we* want them to have, not base our treatment plan upon *their* desired outcomes. I use the phrase, "If you were my sister/brother, here's what I would do…" with patients, but only with their permission when they ask me, "What do you recommend?" You need to think about what is running through the mind of your patients.

- What keeps her up at night?
- What is his biggest concern about dental treatment?
- Why is she putting off dental care you were certain she was ready to start?
- What struggles is he having at home?
- What is her busy schedule like with work and kids on the go?

If you start thinking of your patient as a real person who doesn't live in a dental bubble like you do, you'll gain some invaluable perspective. Your job is much more about psychology and communication than it is about dental care. If you don't want to work on these areas, I suggest you go into hospital dentistry where you can work only on fully sedated patients. But if you want to transform the lives of your patients and team members, you'll need a lot of continuous training and education on PSYCHOLOGY and COMMUNICATION.

Today's consumers are more informed than ever, and many of your patients have already made up their minds about the treatment or outcomes they want BEFORE they walk through your doors. Right or wrong, "Dr. Google" has great influence on your patients as consumers are doing more research on their own than ever. I've had patients come running into my practice seeking dental care because they read something about gum disease and how it links to the rest of our body, or about oral cancer. It wasn't anything I did; it was how they felt at the time and the reassurance they wanted for their restless mind.

Dental schools do a great job of preparing us clinically for practice. Even though most of us leave school feeling like we still have so much to learn in dentistry, I've realized many of the principles I was taught at Virginia Commonwealth University's Dental School, as well as my CE courses and my undergraduate training, have come back to apply to caring for my patients. Clinical care isn't the biggest challenge we face - **the hardest hill to climb in growing your practice is getting and keeping patients.**

You have probably realized this as you've gained clinical experience as well. Where dental schools fail us is in learning real, direct and personalized communication with our patients. You don't learn a lot about empathy, case acceptance or how to run a practice in those four years. We received one week of "practice management" near the end of our final semester of dental school, and it was essentially an optional class that was poorly attended. There just isn't time built into our curriculum to learn how to run and grow a private practice. It's difficult enough to get through the clinical aspects of dentistry in those four fast-paced years that just cruise by. So I'm sharing with you these time-tested principles that I've learned and with which I've built successful systems in my own practice, so that you can do the same.

Why we buy

As Americans, we absolutely LOVE to buy things--we just have to be SOLD on them. In a February 2020 article featured in the *Wall Street Journal* online, a story from early 1950 was described about how, at that time, America had launched into the next phase of a buying-happy nation. "New York City financial executive Frank McNamara and his attorney Ralph Schneider had dinner at the Major's Cabin Grill Restaurant on 33rd St. in Manhattan," the article stated. "When the check came, Mr. McNamara handed the waiter a small paper Diners' Club card and asked to charge the bill. After a year of preparation by the two men, the first charge-card transaction had taken place."

In my experience, payment plans and patient financing are a must today. More than half of Americans have less than $400 in savings, according to the Federal Reserve. Sixty percent of Americans are living paycheck to paycheck, and approximately 20 percent of them are dead broke. That means 80 percent of your neighbors and potential patients are in financial trouble or close to it. You need to offer a better way to help these good people.

Just remember to only offer payment plans and financing to those with good credit. Without at least a "soft credit" check, many patients could borrow money from you that they'll never pay back. In the early years of practicing, I was duped by people with good intentions who would say, "I have bad credit, but I'll pay you back." Unfortunately, the dental bill is at the bottom of their priority list. There are state and non-profit resources for people who are in a bad place financially, and you should help plug them in with the right resources. You should also offer a "charity day" in your practice once a year to give back. Just keep business and charity separate. You must pay your lab, team and your suppliers; you can't afford to have more than 2.5 percent in bad collection accounts.

I was once opposed to payment plans, thinking, "You pay in full at McDonald's and the grocery store when you buy. Why should we be different?" Well, I have learned that we are different for two reasons. One, our average transaction sizes in dentistry are much higher than the average transaction at a restaurant. Two, patients are expecting this expense. Their treatment also takes months to complete.

We can do much better as a profession

The average dental practice has between 38 and 50 percent case acceptance of patient treatment plans. That means half or more of the cases of diagnosed gum disease, dental decay, worn teeth from bruxism and malocclusion goes untreated. This increases the number of teeth that must later be removed or replaced. **We, as a profession, can do better for our patients!**

A May 2020 *Dentaltown* magazine survey reported the following about case acceptance in many practices, regarding how confident doctors were in presenting treatment plans to patients:

- 52 percent said they were very confident
- 41 percent said they were somewhat confident
- 4 percent said they were not very confident
- 3 percent said they have a treatment coordinator or other team member present treatment to patients

How confident is that? No wonder the average practice has only 38 to 50 percent case acceptance for treatment. Forty-seven percent of the respondents had somewhat to nearly zero confidence in presenting. That's an uphill battle. Without this confidence, your patients will delay, say no, or go somewhere else altogether. You have to have confidence and not be forceful or pushy at the same time.

Here's how we've managed to consistently maintain our case acceptance by 45 percent, or above the national average, without slashing our fees or signing up for every insurance plan under the sun. This is very possible, and you can do the same, attracting better patients this way.

Create mapss for boosting your case acceptance

We use a system we have fine tuned over the years we call our Case Acceptance MAPSS. This is discussed more fully in our MAPSS Case Acceptance System (which is not included here), but I'll provide you with an overview so you can implement some of the basics today. MAPSS stands for:

    M - Make your way down the staircase

    A - As a team, make a decision together

    P - Plan the start date

    S - Step 1

    S - (optional, when needed) - Scale back the treatment plan for patients who aren't ready for all or some of your recommended care

Here is a quick overview of our MAPSS treatment planning system. We have used this to consistently increase our case acceptance, while simultaneously building the trust of more patients and being able to offer options without overwhelming our patients. It also helps you gain credibility because those select patients (usually 5 to 20 percent) for whom you can't find a solution will naturally weed themselves out. Not only does this save face for you, but it puts you in a better light and provides you the opportunity to refer these patients to somewhere better suited for them, while you take the higher road of ethically treating people the right way.

As you discuss options, always start with **M: Make your way down the staircase.** Start with your best and highest cost option first. Even if you don't think they will accept it or that it's the best option for your patient, they deserve to know what is available. Even if now isn't the time for them to go with the "premium" option, they may want to do it later. Many of your patients who can't afford or aren't ready mentally for your best options have friends and family who are, so don't cut yourself short and, most importantly, don't pre-judge or assume they want the cheapest option. The best option (which is not necessarily the most expensive) is at the top of your staircase. Start there and work your way down until your patients start to ask more questions and display body language that tells you that you are in the right zone for them.

You should confidently provide your patients with a ballpark cost. Many providers are not comfortable with this, but you have to learn to master it as it's key to demonstrating confidence in your service. You are paid for who you are more than what you do. People want to work with someone they trust, and transparency is key to that. I've been giving costs since I graduated dental school. I wasn't always consistent at it, and I have streamlined my process over the years. Don't worry about what insurance covers, or payment plans - that's the job of your treatment coordinator. You simply need to float the top line number in the direction of your patient and see how they respond to it. You should also give each patient a written estimate of their total responsibility (including what it would be if insurance doesn't pay) and have them sign the estimate prior to treatment.

One of the biggest trust breakers I have witnessed within dental practices is giving patients inaccurate estimates, or telling them "we'll bill you later" and then the patient is shocked when they receive the bill. They will forever believe you messed up if you operate in this way. Always be transparent and make a decision as a three-person team: the patient, your treatment coordinator or team member, and you.

Help your patients understand that the total cost of care is **their responsibility**, not just the estimated cost after insurance. As the dentist/provider, you shouldn't even discuss percentages or copays for insured patients. Leave that part to your treatment coordinator or billing manager. Simply give rough estimates and always round up if needed. That way, as you come down the staircase, it sheds a better light on you and your team as this typically brings the cost down, not up.

Remember that 40 percent or more of your potential patients are uninsured, so don't assume everyone has insurance, either. Many times this group includes some of your best, long-term patients who truly value the care you are giving to them. Your team should ask, "Are you insured or self-pay?" when greeting a new patient, so that the patient doesn't feel it's better to have insurance or to not have it. Show no biases. Be indifferent to insurance, and instead focus your energy on communication and treatment with your patients.

Once your patients agree on a ballpark cost verbally, move to **A: As a team make a decision together**. This is where you iron out the details of your treatment plan. This is where you include the team member(s) who will be scheduling and setting up payment options for your patient to flush out any major concerns they may have. Remember fear, anxiety or perceived lack of need are commonly unspoken objections, so be sure to be direct.

When your patient has verbally acknowledged what they have accepted, move to **P: Plan the start date.** Ask, "Would you like to take care of this today if we have time, in order to save you a trip?" Same-day dentistry has been a huge boost to our practice since day one, and most importantly, your patients really appreciate it.

Even if you aren't sure if you have time to do the treatment today, ask anyway. It helps to flush out any final objections. This is an exception to the open-ended question rule, because you aren't asking them if they want to have the treatment done at all (which could easily solicit a "no" or a negative, closed-ended response), you're simply asking if they'd like to have it done today. If you feel that's too forward, you can modify it to, "Would you like to have this done today, or would you prefer to come back?" If they take the latter option but don't schedule, you have a break in your system no matter how you justify it to yourself. At the very least, you should set up a phone call follow-up. If they aren't a good fit, you should be referring them to someone else at this point, and removing them from your active treatment plan tracking list, so that this doesn't count against your statistics.

Next you'll work your way to **S: Step 1.** This is where you do something to get the ball rolling today. This helps solidify your plan, map out expectations and scheduling, and finish generally consenting for treatment. It could be making impressions, paying an initial investment, or taking x-rays. You want to do something to give value to your patient, save them a trip, help them feel better, and congratulate them on their decision.

Finally, if you get someone who is receptive but then cannot start ideal treatment, you can use the final **S: Scale back (optional, as needed).** This tool will help you to offer a less ideal, but better than nothing treatment. Reassure your patient that other patients have chosen this option as well, so as to not make them feel embarrassed or like they are letting you down. Usually this final S is utilized for patients who cannot afford treatment or do not have credit for financing, but it can also be used for patients who are not able to receive certain treatments due to medical conditions or time restraints.

The MAPSS process will take some practice with your team, as well as role play and fine-tuning. But I'm confident this will boost your case acceptance, and your retention of patients as they discover how transparent you are and how much you care. Carefully considered and planned communication will effectively eliminate most of your problems or potential issues along the way.

Follow up - follow up - follow up

As dentists and practice owners, most of us are Type-A "perfectionists." The problem with this is that we are susceptible to "analysis paralysis." When this phenomenon holds us back, we take too long to act, or may not even act at all, on powerful ideas or changes that can have exponential effects on growing our practices.

An example of this could be adding another doctor, hygienist, or personal assistant that could make your life easier and increase your production by 20, 30 or even 100 percent! The days of a three or four day a week practice are long gone, for the most part. People want an office that suits their needs, not one that suits only your needs. Plus, you can't be closed for four to seven days per week and let your practice sit idle. It's difficult to cover your expenses that way.

Adding more providers and team members, within an acceptable team member efficiency range and payroll budget, will also allow you to expand your reach, in the form of these important areas:

- Expanded hours
- Same-day treatment
- Expanded in-office treatments
- Internal referrals
- Better use of fixed expenses (you're already paying rent or a mortgage; you might as well use the space)

Another great example is creating a follow-up system for contacting your patients by phone, email and letter. It is estimated that people buy after they've had seven to 21 contacts with a business. If you present an implant treatment plan and your patient isn't ready yet, are you following up with them? (Oh yeah, and just one follow-up phone call doesn't count. You need a multi-step follow-up system.) Or are you allowing them to go back out into the world and "Google" other options to replace you? If you aren't following up, you may be missing out on $3,000 to $50,000 in restorative, cosmetic or implant cases left and right.

If you follow the data and research behind this powerful principle, you will see that 80 percent or more of your monthly collection revenue often comes from patients who've been in contact with you seven to 21 times. These contacts could be through word of mouth, recare, seeing you on Facebook, hearing you speak at a local school, or being long-time patients who truly feel that you care about them. Most of the time, people haven't developed enough trust to hand over large amounts of money, time, and commitment when you first meet. Yet, you may still wonder why your patients aren't ready to accept your recommendations. You **must** build trust and pursue it with follow-up. <u>Follow up, follow up, follow up!</u>

I'm a big believer in the ***relentless pursuit of perfection***, but I also must remember that I can't be perfect, and neither can my team members. Neither can you, no matter how hard you may try. Always strive to increase and improve, but enjoy your journey at the same time. As the saying goes, "It's about the journey, not the destination." If you can't be happy with what you are doing now, you probably won't be happy when you get "there" either.

One year on our anniversary, my wife and I snow-hiked to Lake Blanche near Brighton, UT in Big Cottonwood Canyon. It's about a six-mile round-trip hike. We went late, in the very early spring, so there was still a fair amount of snow on the mountain. Just a few miles up the road at one of the ski resorts, they average 500 inches of snow each year and have some of the most popular mountain terrain around.

At the top of the hike, when we reached the lake, we discussed how being on the hike and the exercise that comes with the climb up and down is what we were most excited for, more so than actually getting to the lake.

Remember to be patient and enjoy the journey on the way up. You'll never hit 100 percent, but always pursue it relentlessly and celebrate your wins along the way. Don't forget about your patients, and capitalize by retaining your patients with a multi-step, multimedia, and most importantly, consistent follow-up system.

Tracking is the key to getting better and maximizing your ROI

You may discover that **the #1 thing you can do to grow your practice is to track your results** daily, weekly, monthly, quarterly, and yearly. These are called KPIs, a term originally coined as key performance indicators. We call them key practice indicators, because in dentistry, we are blessed to be in the business of serving and helping people with both their wants and their needs of a winning smile. Get your team on board and track the daylights out of everything you do. We have added more tracking over the years and continually instill in our practice more areas of tracking. When your team members begin to see how important they are and how they are impacted, you'll see your results go up without spending another dollar on marketing or investments.

Most practices I speak with have no tracking or very poor tracking in place. Many dentists and specialists will say, "That doesn't work" or "We tried that"; however, these are usually emotionally based claims and not actual measured results. I've been surprised several times at marketing strategies that actually performed very well, even though we thought them to be laggard. I've also had marketing strategies that we thought were winners that actually tracked poorly, so we learned from them and dropped them from our mix. I love the quote by W. Edwards Deming, who said, "In God we trust; all others bring data." Just like a dental procedure, you need the statistics and data in your study to prove it if really worked or not.

When we started tracking, we had just four or five weekly metrics we tracked, then it grew to what we called the "Bien 10." (Although I'm not anywhere near fluent, bien means "well" in Spanish and it rhymes well with the number ten). If you do well in these areas, you'll have a fantastic growing practice! Just like my belief that all good things come from up above, these metrics are at the top of your funnel that leads to a thriving, growing practice.

Here are the "Bien 10" metrics I suggest you start tracking TODAY, delegating appropriate areas to your team members:

1. New patients
2. Referrals
3. Doctor production
4. Hygiene production
5. Collections
6. Case acceptance
7. Team member retention
8. Charity
9. Accounts receivable
10. Accounts payable

Track these KPIs (key practice indicators) and hold your team members accountable for them on a weekly basis. You should meet with your team once a week to discuss these, identifying areas that need strengthening, identifying what is working well, and then making action items to conquer them, improve them, and execute your RMAP (Relationship Marketing Action Plan). You'll also want to put someone in charge of tracking accounts payable to ensure that your vendors and suppliers are paid on time and treated fairly. These are key relationships we often overlook in our practices, but they are critical to your efficiency and on-time delivery of dental treatment. Remember to: follow up, track, follow up, track, and **repeat**.

On a monthly basis, you should track many more metrics, including over-the-counter vs. insurance collections, open hours of hygiene, etc. Meet once a quarter to review current goals and outcomes, and to set goals for the next quarter. We call these "ROCKS," based on principles taught by Stephen M.R. Covey in his books, *First Things First* and *The 7 Habits of Highly Effective People* (you should definitely read these books if you haven't). As you measure, your practice will grow and your team members will find satisfaction and skill-building challenges in measuring and monitoring. You will find that team members will shoot too high and too low on their goals sometimes, especially in the beginning. You will, too. You have to let them "skin their knees" to learn; you can't micromanage to the point of not letting them learn for themselves. Even if you know the answer, there are times when you have to hold your tongue and let them learn, stretch and grow individually and as a team.

Your job is to be a leader, to stay positive, but also to help them understand WHY you measure these key practice indicators, and that relationships with people are #1 in your book. Always calibrate these KPIs against your core values, and your team will understand the culture in your office and your values.

One area I caution you against is comparing yourself to other offices. Use the most successful practices as examples and resources, but only measure against your best previous months. Use your current KPIs as your baseline and plan as a team how you will grow from there.

There is a great story illustrating the concept of the "grass is always greener," as told by classic author Earl Nightingale, which I will paraphrase here:

Two farmers were constantly complaining about their farms--finding fault in the smallest things and standing on a hill every day, gazing at how great the other farms around them were. One day, the two farmers decided to trade farms, believing that this would solve all of their problems. As soon as they did so, they went up to the hills of their newly claimed farms and gazed out at how great the other farms around them were.

Be grateful for what you have. We live in the best country on earth in which to own a business, with the freedom to practice and to operate how we choose within the boundaries of our ethics and state laws. Compare your growth to your existing practice and learn from your experiences in order to move forward.

Give what you want to receive

Now, more than ever, it's critical as practice owners that we are in the business of giving more value to our patients and team members. Currently, we are right in the trenches of a national crisis. No one knows for certain what will happen next. But what we do know is that major changes are headed our way, both during and after this historical time.

Every time a correction happens, there is a shift: a shift in time, money, effort, trends, and the way we think about our careers and our day-to-day lives. It is a vital time to build and keep the trust of our patients and team members.

As practice owners, it's easy to get caught up in getting credit for how much time and effort we put into a procedure. Most dental professionals are very much in a "what do I get paid per hour" mentality. But this is quite short-sighted. What you should be most concerned with is, how much value do you deliver to the marketplace and to your patients? **What do you give before you receive?** It's how you overdeliver on your services that creates patients you retain, refer and pay on time.

In his fantastic book, *Overdeliver,* author Brian Kurtz states that business is all "about playing the long game." It's not about how much you can get from your patient in one day; it's about how well the relationship will work for both parties in the long run. Kurtz also has a great formula that he calls the "100-0" principle, where, when you give something special to someone, you give 100 percent of your effort and expect nothing in return.

"Shark Tank" co-host Daymond John stated in the March 2020 edition of *Inc.* magazine, "You can't play at being kind or decent or grateful - people will see right through you." In his book, *Powershift,* he describes this as giving three times the value before you ask for anything in return, such as working through dinner three times before asking his employees to do so.

You must give before you receive. It's the Cialdini principle of reciprocity in action. Continually ask yourself, how can I give MORE VALUE to my patient or client?

If your patients don't feel you're giving enough value, they will slowly vanish, until one day you will wonder where all your referral sources and recare patients have gone.

As the stock market was crashing in March 2020, I was struck with a thought about how the curve in financial markets is similar to our relationships with people. In just one instance of failing to follow up, return an important call, or be there when your patient has a major need, you can suffer with a "Relationship Marketing Crash" disaster. If you take too long to react to a call for help, you can lose everything you've worked so hard to build.

It's amazing how all the relationships (or financial gains) that take weeks, months or even years to build up can be crushed with just one bad or neglectful experience. Included in this chapter is the "Relationship Marketing Crash" diagram I developed at Pinecrest Practice Growth to help dental practices and small businesses like yours maximize how you manage these important relationships with your patients.

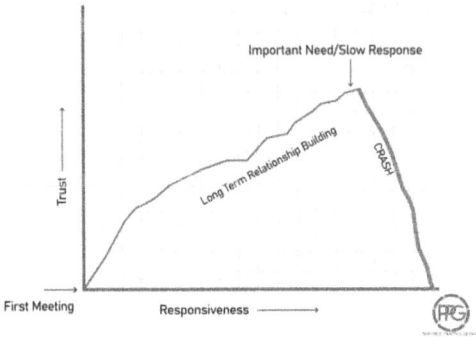

Speed of attack is your #1 defense to keeping solid relationships with your patients. For a great additional resource on this, read Covey's great book titled *The Speed of Trust*. We created a daily follow-up phone tracking sheet that we use in my practice. It can dramatically boost your patient follow-up and case acceptance. Visit yourpracticegrowthbonuses.com for a copy of our daily follow-up phone tracking sheet and other valuable extras mentioned in this book.

Do your patients have real "insurance"?

Insurance premiums for you and your patients keep going up. Are your reimbursements doing the same?

> ***The ONLY reason for you to accept insurance in your practice, in my opinion, is to gain new patients***.

This goes back to the concept you read earlier in the book: "You don't get a patient to do treatment on, you offer treatment to gain trust with a new patient."

Don't think you are doing people a favor or being a "nice person" for discounting your treatment. It does have an effect on your profit, taxes, payroll and long-term goals. ***Insurance is not good or bad, it simply is insurance.*** We are very friendly with insurance in my practice, but we don't let it dictate treatment or the options we give our patients. Dental care is about them - your patient, not about you or the insurance plans you accept. If you accept insurance, then embrace it. Do not knock the hand that feeds you. If you don't, avoid bad-mouthing it. You should be open to accepting it in the future as conditions change.

The cost of accepting insurance continues at each subsequent visit with a happy, loyal patient. In fact, insurance typically costs you more over time. If you accept a 25 percent write-off for each procedure you do, that same write-off will occur every time that patient visits you. Plus, your costs of providing that treatment will rise each year, but your reimbursements will likely barely move up, if at all. According to a February 2020 article from *The Wall St. Journal* online:

> *Prices on nearly every type of insurance are rising, according to insurers and brokers. An exception is workers' compensation, which is highly regulated by states. Excluding workers' compensation, rates for property-casualty insurance sold to businesses rose 6.7% from a year earlier on average in the first three quarters of 2019, on track for the highest annual increase since 2003, according to brokerage Willis Towers Watson.*

What do you really need insurance for? Fires. Disaster. Earthquakes. Catastrophes. The dichotomy is that your patients expect insurance to cover more than it does, and you expect it to cover less. So how do you get around that?

Do you need to join more insurance plans to grow your practice? Or do you need to drop some plans and regain profits? The bottom line is, you need to determine the numbers based on your profit margin and mix of services. If you offer mostly bread-and-butter covered services, you will have a much different equation than if you offer many non-covered services. My practice offers a mix of both covered and non-covered services. So we have determined what our profit margin needs to be and then that makes the decision for us.

If you start accepting more plans, you'll need to be prepared to work more for less, and to be incredibly efficient and cost-saving in your production to make it work. Or, you'll need to get much leaner in the way you and your staff operate.

There isn't a right or wrong answer for you, it's simply your starting point. A 10 to 25 percent write-off may be acceptable to your bottom line, but beware of anything above that. Remember that the average general dental practice has between 60 and 80 percent overhead. Be "insurance friendly" but not "insurance driven" to really do the right thing for your patients. Let them know your stance, and that **preventive dentistry is "real insurance," whether covered or not.** Also remember that 40 percent of your community is uninsured, so provide plans and payment options for them.

Now that you are primed to boost your case acceptance, we'll next discuss WHO should be involved to help you reach those goals. We are blessed to work every day in a profession that is so people-oriented. We get to make lasting differences in the lives of the people for whom we care. These differences can be good or bad, depending on how you approach them. The next three chapters will focus on the "3 Ps" of a growing practice, starting with the Pillar of People.

Chapter 6 Summary:

- The average dental practice has between 38% and 50% case acceptance.

- You can nearly double the average case acceptance rate by following the M.A.P.S.S. System strategies, and the information outlined in this book about what your patient deals with in their day to day life. Solve those problems for them and your case acceptance will go way up.

- Focus on relationship marketing to excel.

- Use marketing and careful case acceptance to build real relationships with your patients.

- Most practices do not follow up constantly or regularly, which is why most practices are at or below the national average for annual production.

- Track everything that you want to improve in your practice, and you will see the trends go in your direction.

Pillar #3: What Is The #1 Asset In Your Practice? It's Your People!

- Chapter Seven -

In the next three chapters you will learn the "3 Ps," which are Pillars 3, 4 and 5 of your 7 Pillars to successful practice growth. These chapters will focus on People, Production, and Place, respectively. We'll start with the People Pillar first, because your team and your patients are your top assets in your practice. Payroll is one of, if not your largest expense (that is actually an investment), so it's critical you manage and monitor your payroll numbers every month. It translates to what we call Team Member Efficiency.

When I graduated from dental school, I thought dental procedures would be the most challenging area of my practice. WRONG! Working with **people is likely to be your biggest challenge**. I would be lying to you if I told you this chapter would magically make all of your problems with people go away. But I will tell you that I will help you learn to recruit the right type of team members and the right type of patients, so that your people problems will be minimized by 80 percent or more! It can be done, but it takes lots of training, follow-up, recalibration and repeat. If you hate doing this, then find someone on your team who would like to take on this responsibility and delegate it to them, but it must be done to have a great team and practice.

There are four main groups of people in your practice network of whom you should be mindful in order to maintain great relationships with them. Continually find ways to grow and nurture these relationships. They can be long-lasting and can benefit you and the other person greatly in the long run. These three groups include:

1. Your team members
2. Your patients
3. Your vendors (including software companies, consultants, accountant, CPA, insurance companies, suppliers, labs, salespeople, etc.)
4. Your community leaders and neighbors

People make life interesting. Stories, events, and real interaction is one of, if not the best, part of what we do in our jobs. One of my first patients ever in practice was a Vietnam vet who had a pre-existing gold crown on either side of his mouth, one with a Swastika on the casting, and the other crown with a Star of David on it. I never saw him much, but he said the story was for another day, and I'm sure it had to do with a graphic experience he had in the war. Although I wouldn't suggest you offer this type of crown to your patients, it was something I'll never forget. I have received countless thank yous, cards of appreciation, wedding and anniversary cards, and video testimonials of story after story from my patients. **This is what I get excited for, and it all comes from having a Relationship Marketing Action Plan** to build up your "relationship deposit account," which is what really matters at the end of the day. Over the years the stories have grown more into care, compassion and healing for my patients, and I'm sure they are a big motivator for you as well.

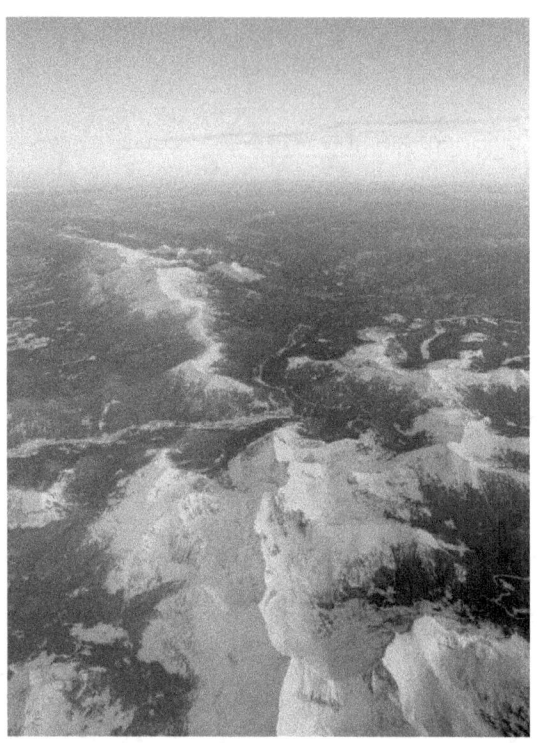

Create a stronger team

I took the photo in this chapter from an airborne view of the Rocky Mountains while traveling to Denver late in October 2019 for a small business conference I attended. It snowed just a couple days before I arrived, and after the two-day event, the Mile High city was forecasted for an early fall 15 inches of snow. Thankfully my flight was out of there before the storm hit.

My kids and I enjoy skiing and snowboarding together. One of my kids rides a snowboard and the other two ski. I've done both sports, but I've been snowboarding for the past 24 years or so and I'd never had a significant injury doing it...until I FELL one January night a few years ago in my home state of Utah. When I heard a big loud "SNAP" sound, I immediately knew it was going to be bad. Instantly I had severe pain and could hardly move my right arm. It was paralyzing - like nothing I'd ever felt before. So what happened...

I dislocated my shoulder on the slopes.

I wish I could brag about some impressive trick I was doing, but I was simply going a little off the cat track and up a small wall jump. Suddenly, I turned wrong, caught my edge in the snow, and next thing I knew, I was headed down the hill, shoulder first into the soft powder. (I'm really becoming a wimp, I guess?) SNAP! I sprang to my feet, hoping that I would be okay. My right arm was numb, and when I tried to move it, I was in extreme pain. My two older kids stopped and said, "Dad, are you okay? You don't seem okay." My racing mind thought that at least my legs were fine and I could have gone down the hill if I had to, even with the injury.

About ten seconds later, I was able to pop my shoulder back in. It's still a little tight, but I've had full range of motion for about nine months now, thanks to some stretching, exercise and laser therapy from the chiropractor. Fortunately, I am left-handed, so I was able to work the entire time. Aside from breaking my arm on my backyard trampoline when I was six, this was the closest call to a broken bone or joint I've had in my lifetime. I consider myself pretty blessed.

Our society and educational system has programmed us that to "fail" is the worst thing we can do. Think about it. Did you ever receive a bad grade in school? Get a speeding ticket? Fail a licensure exam or test? Maybe you have and maybe you haven't, but failing is an opportunity to learn and get better, not a judgment on our intellect or character.

> *"Success consists of going from*
> *failure to failure*
> *without loss of enthusiasm."*
>
> -Winston Churchill

In certain aspects of life, I'm very cautious and careful, but in others, I have no problems taking risks. I love trying new things. The problem with being told that we "failed" is that it can make us hesitant to try out something that can make us better or provide us with an exciting new opportunity.

There's only a slight difference between the spelling of "fall" and "fail." Only one simple letter. But a fail/fall is something we should learn from. I can either quit snowboarding or learn to be more careful (and coordinated!). I'll be back up to the mountain again this winter with my kids, but I'll be taking a new approach to avoid "catching my edge" again.

When managing people, both patients and team members, it's critical that you "bend but don't break." You have to be flexible, but set boundaries on what is okay and what isn't inside your walls.

A year later, my shoulder was not 100 percent, but my muscles became stronger than they had been in a long time. I was working out five to six days per week and training with more weights to increase my shoulder strength more than I ever had before..

If something is sprained or wounded in your practice, address it now to nourish and revive it. If something is broken in your practice, it will take much longer to heal, so be patient. Break the job up into smaller pieces and delegate parts of it to your most eager team members who want to help you.

Do not worship the "Volcano God of Pain." Dr. Jerome Groopman wrote a fascinating book about his eperiences as an oncologist caring for patients and cancer survivors, called, *The Anatomy of Hope: How People Prevail In The Face Of Illness,* In it, he states, "The more you sacrifice, the more (the god of pain) demands until your life contracts, as it has, into a very, very narrow space." Don't feed the bad things going on in your life or practice. Find what drives you, bring in the people who will help you get results, and feed those thoughts and those people to help you move your thermometer to where you want it to be. Use your energy to find solutions to the big problems, and the little ones will work themselves out.

Our educational system tells us we're "wrong" when we fail, but failing once in a while is actually the right thing to do in order for maximum growth and learning to occur. The difference between the losers and the winners is what you do with that information once you've learned from it. It's the same with a CE course that you attend; it is just "interesting information" if you don't implement it into your practice. **Implementation and acting on what you learn is the way to success.**

Focus on PGE: Practice Growth for Everyone. Don't design a profit sharing or incentive system that only benefits you, make one where the whole team gets to join in when you meet or exceed your goals. Use a tiered system to make your incentives challenging yet motivating.

Create your offense with a great defense

Just one bad team member can be toxic to your team and culture. It may be inadvertent, or a result of personal issues outside of work, but don't let a laggard team member who doesn't buy into your values and work ethic infiltrate your team.

I've learned this the hard way!

Have you ever hung on to someone too long, hoping they would do better because you didn't want to fire them and didn't want to find a replacement? Sound familiar?

Take a note from successful sports teams: **often the "best offense is a good defense."** You must defend and maintain the health of your team and culture. When you hang on to a team member who just isn't in it, they are defeating the morale of your best team members. Listen to them.

I'll share a quick thought from the book, *How to Make Money in Stocks,* by the founder of Investors Business Daily, William O'Neil. He is referring to the glory days of the Brooklyn Dodgers:

> *"In the game of baseball, the combination of pitching and fielding represent the defensive side of the team and probably 70 percent of the game. It's almost impossible to win without them."*

The same idea holds true for your practice. Defend and reinforce your core values and principles of service, or die. **Do not accept complacency or stagnation. Instead, demand constant personal and team improvement** (including yourself - do not be a hypocrite), and lead by example.

At the same time, don't expect perfection. In certain military operations, having 70 percent of the needed information is enough to act upon. Eighty percent gets you a B in school. Good enough is good enough in most cases, so don't be overly-perfectionist. Instead emphasize the good things your team does, and work on taking the 80 percent achievements to an 88 percent score, then to 95 percent. Always shoot for the highest score possible and constantly push your goals to the next level, but don't be disappointed when you fall below 100 percent. Celebrate your wins and write a "WOW!" card or thank you note to your team members.

Get rid of toxic influences

In your patients with gum disease, just one family of toxic bacteria can contaminate the whole mouth. It does you absolutely zero good to have just one bad apple on your team. In fact, it does the opposite: it actually damages and weakens the attitude, motivation, and culture of your entire team when you allow bad team members to be hired or to stay with your team. Examples include:

- Team members who always complain about their pay structure, no matter where it's at. (Throwing more money at someone or something is never a good solution for a problem.)
- Team members who are not going to learn or improve their skills or communication habits.
- Team members who are always late.
- Team members who do not meet deadlines.
- Team members who always have an excuse.
- Team members who are negative and say things like, "That won't work for us." Or they may say, "We can't do that here."
- Team members who require exponentially more time and training than the rest of your team, sucking up the valuable time of your best team members.

You need to remove these people from your surroundings promptly and efficiently. If they are honest with themselves or are truly seeking to become better, they will appreciate your candor and you'll be doing them a big favor by helping them have a better future. They may not even realize how negative they are being and the damage that negativity is causing. Just like an abscessed tooth, you need to treat this infectious situation quickly to relieve the pressure. Most practice owners do not want to have this confrontation, but it only gets harder the longer you wait.

In his *New York Times* bestseller, *The Book of Secrets: Unlocking the Hidden Dimensions of Your Life*, Dr. Deepak Chopra shares how to develop a better outlook on the persons with whom you surround yourself. He recommends developing this kind of attitude:

"I will no longer bring my problems to anyone who wants to leave me alone. It's not good for me. They don't want to help, so I will not ask them to... I will share my problems with those who want to help me. I will not

reject genuine offers of assistance out of pride, insecurity, or doubt. I will ask these people to join me...and make them a bigger part of my life... I will put distance between myself and those who want to hurt me. I do not have to...guilt-trip them, or make them the cause of my self-pity. But I can't afford to absorb their toxic effect on me and if that means keeping my distance, I will."

Your team will respect you much more if you establish this type of culture in your practice, where you surround yourself with winners and people with a can-do, positive attitude. On the flipside, Dr. Chopra talks about studies showing that when teachers are told in advance that a certain student is exceptionally bright, that student typically "performs much better in class even if this election was random." Think positively about team members and how you can lift them up to a higher level of development and to personal goal-setting, and remove those who are not willing to work with you as a team.

Learning to train and develop as a team

It's important that you meet with your team regularly and practice communication. I find it interesting that professional athletes, such as NBA players, practice every day during the season to perform in just a couple of games each week. Yet most dental practices go straight to "game time" (treating patients and being busy with your day), with very little thought, role play, or practice beforehand. *How do you get your "daily practice" in with your team?*

One way for you to tackle this is with a Monday meeting held each week. You should also plan out daily practice, where your team members are quizzed on a couple key points about their role in the office. We call these our "Foundational 14" key parts of a position. They are made up of the 20 percent most important principles to any one position in the office (80/20 rule), such as dental hygienist or treatment coordinator. You can make flash cards or a printed Word document with these in them. It typically takes two to two and a half weeks for a new, full-time team member to complete learning these principles, and that becomes their initial certification. They are writing down answers, rather than you telling them everything they need to know. Help them feel confident, but don't do the research and work for them. We use Google Drive (drive.google.com) for storing all of our systems, but you could also have a printed binder as well. Each of our team members is required to recertify on the "Foundational 14" every six months.

After someone is certified or recertified, we hang up a Gold Star Certification sheet in a mounted photo frame in our hallway to show off what our team members have learned. You'll be surprised at how much pride your team members will take in this accomplishment. It also keeps them accountable to your systems and practice culture.

You should plan periodic review days and team training days throughout the year as well. One hour of good planning can save you two to ten hours of wasted time later, and can also do amazing things for your productivity. Besides our Monday meeting each week (which lasts for 70 minutes) we also hold a review day ten to 14 days before the end of each quarter. During this quarterly meeting, we recap the current quarter, discuss how to finish it strong, include any adjustments that need to be made, and plan our goals for the next quarter.

Research has demonstrated that **most of what you learn is forgotten within a day or so unless you write it down and implement it**. You may see some great restorative cases or clinical tips, and get excited to do them yourself. Then, you may debate on whether or not these cases or tips will work for you. Before you know it, 75 percent of what you have learned is forgotten, usually within 24 hours - unless you implement it immediately. (Even if you're a genius, you will still forget many important things quickly. Look up the "Forgetting Curve" research from Cal State University for more info on this fascinating topic.)

Bad vs. Good communication will cause (or eliminate) 99 percent of your problems

Earlier in this book, I wrote about communication and how it is rarely or barely taught to us in formal education, but how vital it is to the success of a practice or business. Some time ago, one of our treatment coordinators and I were invited to a dental treatment seminar in Las Vegas. The group discussed different types of dental and orthodontic treatment, and how we could better serve our patients and team members at the office.

In a sense, the seminar was all about communication. Although this wasn't the specific topic, I am a strong believer that nearly all of our problems in our personal and professional relationships can be prevented with great communication.

I'm not talking about sending more text messages (I'm not a big texter anyway - just ask my wife, it drives her nuts) or doing more talking. I'm talking about really working to understand each other and the people we are around every day. **I sincerely believe that good communication can eliminate 99 percent of your problems**. Here's why:

Communication is like a three-legged chair:

Leg 1 - Effective delivery of information

Leg 2 - Behavior of the recipient

Leg 3 - Retention of information

Professor Albert Mehrabian at UCLA ran a study back in the 1960s about communication. He later published a book about this and more, entitled *Nonverbal Communication*. Here's what his research discovered:

55 percent of effective communication is in the non-verbal exchange.

38 percent of effective communication is in the verbal exchange.

7 percent of effective communication is in the words you say.

The research further found that there are five behaviors you go through when you are making a decision, such as whether to purchase something:

1. Problem recognition
2. Information gathering
3. Evaluation
4. Purchase decision
5. Post-purchase decision

Finally, as described by Dr. L.D. Rosenblum in his book, *See What I'm Saying,* and from the website, Velvet Chainsaw, all communication is received through your five senses: sight, sound, smell, taste and touch. It's important to understand which of the senses are more dominant to you and those you work with, as we all process and value certain ways of communication differently. They concluded that dividing amongst your senses, **you retain**:

83 percent of what you SEE

11 percent of what you HEAR

3.5 percent of what you SMELL

1.5 percent of what you TOUCH

1 percent of what you TASTE

In summary, this is why visuals such as presentations, video and pictures are such powerful tools. If, according to the UCLA research, effective communication is 55 percent non-verbal and 38 percent verbal, this equals 93 percent of communication through sound and sight.

Add to that retention of information, based on Dr. Rosenblum, which teaches us that 83 percent of your senses are based upon what you see, and 11 percent are based upon what you hear, this equals 94 percent - again, communication that is based on sight and sound.

Finally, for you math geeks like me, averaging 93 percent and 94 percent gives you 93.5 percent, that's an A! This is a very high percentage strategy to eliminate your problems and boost your case acceptance from your patients. Remember, only seven percent of communication was based upon the actual words said. This is why the old saying that "actions speak louder than words" still rings true today.

Perhaps this is why I distinctly remember all of the dumb things my friends did as teenagers trying to impress each other, or all of the things I learned in high school health class that scared the life out of me!

Recently, I read an article about new shoes that are controlled by an app, so that you can be glued to your phone while walking down the street, and the app will tell your shoes which way to turn. MRI scans done on the brains of millennials (I am just barely a millennial, so I can speak from experience) found that opening a digital message is much less impactful than opening a real letter, or interacting with printed media such as a book. Technology definitely has its place, but I don't think it will ever replace REAL, one-on-one communication. Remember this next time you are communicating with your spouse, team members and patients.

Use the M.A.P.S.S. Case Acceptance tool to leverage communication by understanding the tone and body language of your patients. This will show how much you care and help them accept treatment that is in line with the outcome that they want.

Apply the "2/1 rule of communication"

As mentioned earlier, you can never be too thorough with your communication, in my experience. This is why I developed something I call the 2/1 rule of communication. This rule is defined as follows:

For every one question or request received from a patient team member or vendor you should follow up and respond with at least two methods of communication.

For example, if a patient calls you after hours and leaves a message that they would like a call back due to a chipped tooth or a question on their bill, call them back. If you don't speak with them in person, leave a voicemail. Afterward, send them a text message or email stating that you returned their call, and include your name and best method of contact to be reached. Keep in mind your local and state laws regarding HIPAA for the types of communication you can use. Typically, text messages and email are okay, as long as you don't share sensitive information in the communication. This illuminates the problem of, "Oh, I called her back and left a message" that the patient may or may not have received. When you use at least two methods of communication, such as letter, postcard, phone call, voicemail, text message, email, it leaves very little room for someone to say you never responded to them.

Set achievable but challenging goals

Each of us starts out on a goal with energy and motivation. It's exciting to have a new, big goal with a fresh start ahead of you. So why do we so often fail to hit the target? Why do we lose motivation halfway through? A new study from Science Direct, which uncovered the effort-reward challenge at the intersection of neuroscience and behavioral science, offers a simple but useful insight about the failure to reach goals. It centers on the disconnect between our decision-making focus before we start pursuing a goal, and our focus after we begin working towards our goal.

The research started with this hypothesis: when we set out to achieve a goal, our focus is on the reward. We envision getting the reward, and how we'll feel when we conquer the goal, and that launches us into action. The problem is, once we begin, we come face-to-face with what's really required to reach the goal, and our focus shifts from reward to effort. Here's the kicker: instead of refocusing on the reward, we stay focused on the effort. The research found that:

The more you focus on effort,
the more likely you are to fail.

The results of the experiments were consistent for both physical and mental effort:

> *The amount of the financial reward influenced how the participants chose their effort-reward combinations, as expected. But when they started the work, their performance was determined by how much effort reaching the reward was really going to require, regardless of how much money was at stake.*

Never assume that someone else has taken care of something or someone. If no one has been identified as the team member in charge to take care of that person or problem, always clarify. Have the team member repeat it back to you, or, better yet, to your patients. **Just like drinking water, communication can never be too clear.**

A few years ago when our oldest son was just two, my wife and I were picking up some items in IKEA and he got lost inside the store. Here's how it happened.

We split up, intending to go to different areas of the store in order to finish more quickly. We both needed to grab some big boxes, and we were also in a rush to get to our next appointment on our schedule that day. (Plus I just hate shopping, so I always feel in a rush at any store.) We briefly spoke about who would be keeping our son, Judson, by their side. Of course, she thought I was taking him and I thought she was taking him. We didn't clarify. Because of this, he wasn't sure either, and he became lost in the store. It was a scary life lesson, but fortunately, he taught us something very valuable that we will never allow to happen again with him, or with our other children. From this experience, we learned how to better communicate with each other and with him.

WHAT DO YOU ABSOLUTELY LOVE TO DO?

Take a moment to think about what kinds of activities or opportunities get you really excited. What do you really LOVE to do?

What gets you out of bed in the morning?

Who in your circle of influence do you love to work with or be around?

Do you love your job as a dentist?

How do you feel about your practice, patients, and team?

What hobbies do you really enjoy?

What recreational activities do you look forward to participating in?

These are all important aspects of your life to recognize and reflect on, not just for what and who they are, but for your mental and physical health. If your answer is no, or you can't come up with an answer to any of these, you need to make a change in your life.

If I really had to do it, I could work more than I do (not that it would be healthy to do so). I especially enjoy working on the practice, because I love being in the "lab" of testing new ideas to grow my team, make our patient experience better, and find new ways to hit our goals with marketing. This is what gets me excited to jump out of bed each morning.

The question to ask yourself is, how do you show your appreciation to those around you?

One thing that makes a big difference in your practice is sending "TLC" cards to your patients and vendors. TLC stands for "tender loving card," and it's a simple, handwritten thank you note. Send these out every week. In fact, I suggest you make it a requirement that your team members mail out at least three of these every month as part of their job requirement and a monthly incentive for payroll check. If you don't do this already, you will begin to notice the gratitude that your team members have for your best patients and for each other. In a world of digital communication, handwritten notes are becoming more scarce. They really do help you stand out and express gratitude for the people in your sphere of influence.

It's vitally important that you set the example as well. In my leadership planner, I have a section each week where I will write a list of people to whom I will send a TLC. You may also send gifts or write notes for your team members to show your appreciation to them. You can get a card that says "Wow!" and tape a dollar bill to it. Then, write a note about something you appreciate about a team member and put it in their locker or inbox. We get those silver or gold one-dollar coins and tape them to the premade cards, and then I put one in an employee's locker each week. They appreciate it, and it helps to remind me about all of the work that goes into taking care of our patients. If you aren't doing this already, you should. Not only is it a huge morale booster for your team, but you will notice your efficiency and productivity go up, because your team members will feel the culture of your office and realize that what they do at work goes far beyond a paycheck.

Just like your recare patients, if someone doesn't hear from you at least a couple of times per year, the relationship will fade. Think about friends you haven't heard from or seen in a long time. Can you really say you have a solid relationship with them? Probably not.

You can create a simple index card system, which I call "Relationship Recare." I took this concept from some direct mail research that says if your customers (or patients) don't hear from you every six months, then they are just as likely to find a new dentist, dry cleaner, hairdresser, etc. who reaches out or markets to them.

This is how you lose patients. It's our responsibility to reach out to them, because most don't care about or think about dental care nearly as much as we do.

This is why you should also have a reactivation plan for patients who haven't been in your office for 181+ days. It's not that they have forgotten about you; they get busy, just like you do. Reach out to them and show how much you care. Do the same with your neighbors, friends, mentors, employees, family members, etc. Send a TLC card or make a phone call periodically and see how much your relationships grow. (FYI, for team members I do this at least monthly, or more, but every six months is a *MINIMUM* guideline for you to adhere to for growing the strength of your relationships.)

For more tips on creating a Relationship Recare system for your life and team members, visit www.yourpracticegrowthbonuses.com

Fail to succeed

Due to the Coronavirus panic of March 2020, my weekend plans for an anniversary getaway to Lake Tahoe were cancelled. We were pretty bummed about the adventure we had to put on hold, but knew it was the safer bet. Truthfully, we weren't that concerned about the actual virus, but more concerned about being quarantined away from our kids or stuck on a tarmac somewhere. I hate acting out of fear, and felt that was what we were doing at the time, but we had to put our kids and family first. The news and media were talking like it was doomsday, as the stock market had its largest drop since the 1987 crash. Schools cancelled, churches cancelled, spring breaks were extended on college campuses - with the understanding that they would likely have to finish the semester online.

The Costco near my home had generated $1.2 million in sales on its biggest day during the Christmas season just a few months prior. However, it went on to earn even more--a total of $1.5 million--on March 12, with people lined up to purchase paper products and bulk food.

The first day of our Tahoe trip was going to be practice-related. We were planning to attend an office design tour so that I could extract some ideas to implement in my building that was under construction at the time. I was excited to get some "big picture ideas" and to further develop my long-term plans for my team, my patients and my family.

I strongly believe that there is a reason for everything, even if we can't understand it at the time. I have learned that when one door closes for you, another one opens. I've been frustrated so many times in the past when something didn't work out the way I had planned or hoped. Finally, one day, I decided to always look for the opportunity in a good or bad experience. I have always been a glass-half-full kind of guy, but I also have a short temper about certain things, and have let that get in the way too many times. But I have learned that being short-sighted leads to wasted time and energy.

During the snowy season in northern Utah, we sometimes see "winter storm warning" broadcast on news and TV. These storms often end up producing just a few inches of snow, which is not a big deal for us here, because we are used to and typically prepared for it. However, information like this is likely harmful to the sales of your local car wash, restaurants, or movie theaters. Weather leads to some cancellations in your practice, too.

Through the many ups and downs of life's adventures, I've learned that the quicker I can turn "skinning my knees" into squeezing out the valuable lessons and using them as a stepping stone for improving my life plan, the easier it is to find the nuggets of wisdom in an experience.

John Maxwell calls these "learning opportunities" and terms it "failing forward." I once read that in business, we have <u>only two outcomes from an event: 1) learning opportunities and 2) success - there are no actual failures</u>. We "fail" at certain things, but we shouldn't label someone as a "failure" based on one static moment in time. Schools are notorious for motivating us out of fear of not failing rather than driving the creative output that can come from the right kind of motivation.

Inspiring real learning is where you should aim your focus for both your team and yourself, individually.

This may sound too idealistic to you, but if you develop this mindset, it sure makes it a lot easier to sleep at night. Some of my biggest failures in the past have totally changed my business and leadership outlook for the better, even though it takes dedicated time to develop. The amygdala is the part of your brain that takes fear and turns it into your body's defense mechanisms. Your prefrontal cortex and hippocampus, on the other hand, are the parts of your brain that develop gratitude and creativity. You can't feed both the fearful parts and the creative parts of your brain at the same time. **Which one are you feeding, developing and growing?**

Plato is quoted as saying, "courage is knowing what not to fear." This is critical wisdom to heed during a viral outbreak, stock market crash or slow month in your practice. Not only does fear make you feel terrible, but it does not allow your creative mind the ability to grow and produce new ideas and systems to build up your practice. Your goals thermometer (we use whiteboard thermometers to measure our goals on a monthly basis) does not fill up based on fear. Simply put:

You can't live in fear of failing and have a life of attainment.

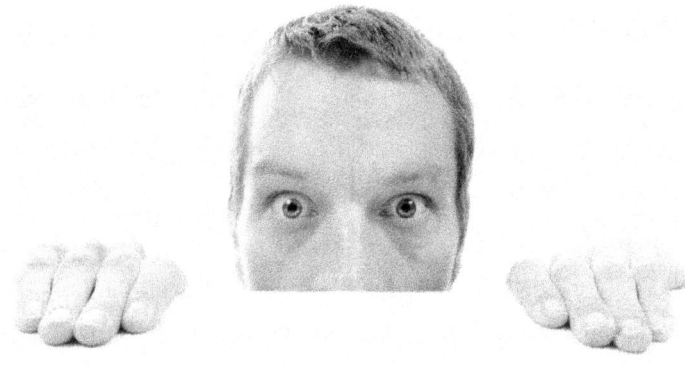

Image source: pixabay.com

Remember to stay ahead of the majority, because as Dan Kennedy says, **the majority is usually wrong**--otherwise the 80/20 rule wouldn't apply, nor would highly productive practices, top athletes, or the most successful people be where they are today. <u>They are the minority</u>. Developing your mind, your education and your team is one of the best ways to avoid living in fear. Instead, learn to live in a mindset of growth and abundance. If the economy zigs, it's time for you to zag. Do the opposite of what most people do if you want to do something exceptionally well. If you have to close for a few days due to unforeseen circumstances, use them as personal days or planning days to boost your morale and inspire bold new ideas to take your team and your practice to the next level.

What are you doing with your spare time?

When you have extra time, how do you spend it? I once heard a saying that goes something like this: "it's not what you do in your nine-to-five job that counts, it's what you do in your spare time that really matters." I've observed the most successful, most productive people plan for time off and plan for relaxation time, but they don't just let it happen. They block out this time in their schedule. In the practice, we refer to this as we must "manage the schedule rather than let the schedule manage us." Never leave anything up to chance, including your personal time, otherwise it won't happen.

In my personal Leadership Planner, I schedule and color code my days by the "3 Ps," which are Personal Days, Planning Days, and Production Days, planned in that order of priority. After studying what other successful business owners do, I have adapted this for running my dental practice. I also produced a similar spiral-bound version of this planner that I give to each of my team members as well. It took hours of my time and working with our graphic designer to create, but it is worth its weight in gold (and it is heavy, over 300 pages' worth of yearly tools).

What are you reading in your personal time, or are you reading at all? One of my favorite activities when I have personal time, including during my workouts, is to read or listen to books. I use the Audible and Audiobooks apps for listening, and have a library of real books (you know, those things printed on real paper) that I continue to add to, as well as a section of my favorites that I reread on an annual basis. When you listen to positive motivation during your workouts, they become much more meaningful, and provide a constant stream of new ideas to implement into your practice.

Some of the best ideas you can gain will be from books completely UNRELATED to dentistry. You live in a dental "thought bubble" that has been around for decades. Sure, some of the old stereotypes are changing, but dentistry has not conventionally been known as a highly-rated, service-oriented industry. It is a doctor-oriented industry, which is important for a good clinical outcome, but it explains why studies have shown that as much as 50 percent of the population has not seen a dentist in the past year. People do business with people that they know, trust and like, and many people do not trust or like going to the dentist.

One of the best books for you to read, then reread and share with your team is by social psychologist Robert Cialdini, titled *Influence: The Psychology of Persuasion*. His follow-up book, *Pre-Suasion,* is also a great read, but *Influence* is still the better read for your dental practice in my experience.

The six principles from this book that he discusses in the book, and that you should implement into your team training to better your patient experience, are:

1. Reciprocity
2. Consistency
3. Social Proof
4. Liking
5. Authority
6. Scarcity

It all starts with how your patients feel when they interact with you. Here's how you can convert these social psychology principles into increasing your "people output" in your practice to accelerate your growth.

Reciprocity is giving BEFORE you ask. When a new or reactivated patient comes to your office, put aside the discussion of insurance or payments until AFTER you have provided your patient with a tour of your office, a consultation, or a gift from your team. Make it about them, not about their insurance or even their teeth. People come first. When you do this, your rewards will be multiplied and your patients will really see how much you care.

Consistency means you provide a repeatable experience for your patients time and time again. They are greeted with a scripted call each time they reach out to you. You respond to any request within 24 hours. They are offered "comfort items" at each visit from a menu that a team member shares with them. You check out the patients the same way each time. Place lip balm on their lips after every appointment. You have to decide which things are the most important to consistently apply to your patient experience, and you should be adding new ones each year to keep it interesting. It will take hours of role play between your team members and meetings to implement it, but the rewards will be great. Just like in sports, a well-trained team and well-practiced game plan leads to a high rate of success.

Social Proof comes in many forms today. You may be using Facebook and Instagram, Google Reviews, Yelp, and doctor-specific sites such as Healthgrades to spread the word about you to your community. YouTube is also a powerful tool for you to use on a regular basis to provide interactive content with your patients. You should take advantage of this free tool to boost the way your patients see you. (By the way, there are some best practices for doing this. Just because it's free, it doesn't mean it doesn't require strategy. If you have questions, reach out to my office and we'll fill you in.)

But don't just limit your social proof to social media. In fact, real people, real testimonials and real before-and-after photos can be much more powerful for your patients and prospects. They are timeless marketing assets - meaning as social media sites come and go, **they will still be relevant to boost your case acceptance and bottom line collections year after year**. Most importantly, you should use social proof to help your patients understand how other patients, just like them, have had great experiences, obtained the results they wanted, or transformed their smile.

Liking is related to the old adage, "people do business with people they know and trust." As video expert Ron Sheetz said, "Attention breeds familiarity and familiarity breeds trust....People are influenced by the direction of things more than the state of things. People want to be wowed." Your patients want to like the person who is working on their smile. They want to like the team who answers your phone and responds in a timely manner to their emails and texts. They want a quick turnaround and want an answer faster than ever, a challenge you'll have to keep up with.

In 2011, Adweek.com reported that our attention spans had decreased on average from twelve minutes to five minutes. Seven years later, attention spans appeared to have become even shorter, as one Google report found that when a page takes more than three seconds to load, 53 percent of site visitors leave. Other research is clueing us in on how this works, and has found that it is probably related to your attention evolving more than anything. There is just so much coming at us all of the time, people are getting pickier about what they read.

Personally, I prefer real books and magazines rather than online content. This a big reason you should be using direct mail and newsletters to reach your patients, not just email. (As of today, email open rates are dropping. Even with your best group patients, you probably won't see much more than a 20 percent open rate on any one email.) You want to find unique ways for your patients to like you and develop a team that they will like as well. This isn't easy, but it is required in today's competitive business and practice environment.

Authority is about how you position yourself. It's not about being a dentist--it's about becoming *the dentist for their needs*. As I mentioned earlier, the "cottage industry" of dentistry has been around for decades, and although it's changing, it has been all about the dentist/doctor-driven practice. Today, you need a team and patient-driven practice. Authority marketing for dentistry is about getting involved in your community, writing helpful articles for your patients, and becoming an expert on topics relevant to your existing patients.

Many patients see you as exactly the same as all other dentists. They think that you use the same composite, the same implants, and the same clear aligners to fix their teeth as everyone else does - UNLESS you give them a reason to think otherwise. As dentistry becomes more commoditized, your prices will be driven down, insurance will dictate your treatment plans, and your profit margins will vanish, unless you customize your treatment plans and offer multiple options to your patients. It's about their needs, not yours, but becoming a local authority in a topic, or even a local hero for a charity you are involved in can be a new patient magnet for growing your practice.

Scarcity means limiting your time in any one given activity. Have you timed your average crown or tooth removal procedure? How long does it take? The same goes for your morning team huddle, your end-of-day checklists and your time for emails each day. You must limit these or they will expand and fill your day with things that are less important and often irrelevant to achieving your big goals. Parkinson's Law teaches us that "work expands to fill the time available for its completion." This goes back to managing your schedule, both personally and professionally. If you don't manage it, your schedule will manage you, so take charge of it today.

With any form of marketing you engage in, use scarcity to limit the deadline or quantity of the offer, and stick to it. If a patient brings in a coupon for a free dinner gift certificate with a paid cleaning after the deadline, what do you do? Still give them the offer? Or play hardball and say "no"? You must stick to your word, but there's a balance. Rather than cave in, still be generous and say, "We wish that (offer name) was still available, but since the deadline expired we are no longer offering that incentive. However, we appreciate you (as a patient, as an on-time patient, as a long-time patient, etc.), and can offer you a (free whitening consultation, bottle of xylitol mouthrinse, etc.) for bringing that offer in and getting your cleaning done today."

Remember, if you don't stick to the deadlines on marketing offers, you won't stick to a deadline with your schedule, and you'll indirectly allow your team and patients to run late, which will increase your stress and hammer your productivity. I've learned this firsthand and have made the mistakes for you, so you don't have to do the same. Leverage these principles to your advantage and plan for success. Your output is a result of your input. Plan ahead and hold your team accountable to the goals you set together!

Use "knockout" rate speed to get growth results

To have perfect vision is to have a perfectly clear understanding of what you see in front of you. A vision for the future of your practice. This includes today's vision, tomorrow's vision, and next year's vision. In the bestselling book, *Traction,* by Geno Wickman, the author provides a powerful insight on how to set a one-year, three-year and ten-year plan. If you don't already, you should create and have these in place for your business, refer to them regularly, and update them annually with your team.

In January 2020, history was made in the UFC Mixed Martial Arts world of sports as Colin McGregor routed Donald "Cowboy" Cerrone with a TKO in 40 seconds. McGregor was like a raging, charging bull and took down the Cowboy with lightning speed. <u>McGregor had a plan and executed it perfectly</u>, and by doing so was rewarded handsomely. He received a guaranteed $3 million just for showing up, but took home an estimated $80 million with all of his payouts, according to CBS Sports. Why does McGregor receive so much money and so much attention? Because:

McGregor is controversial.

McGregor is cocky.

McGregor loves to promote himself and his brands.

McGregor has a trademark "billionaire" walk that goes before him.

Whether you like him or not, he knows how to win. He has a clear vision for his professional career and his company. He had so much confidence going into the fight, that he instantly took over and blindsided the Cowboy in a matter of seconds. Simply put, McGregor knew exactly how to get the result he wanted.

Although you should treat your patients much more respectfully, **the questions for you to ask yourself are:**

Do you know how to get the results you want in your practice?

Do you have a crystal clear vision for your future?

Does your team know what your vision is?

The key to having a growing practice is being able to articulate how to execute your plan. You don't have to be perfect to be a success. I've certainly made more than my share of blunders as I've grown my own practice. But you have to "skin your own knees" and "kiss a few frogs" on the journey to producing a winning formula.

<u>By leaning on the experience and advice of those who are more successful than you, you will make fewer mistakes, save a lot of potentially wasted money, and save yourself a lot of time</u>.

McGregor is probably not your ideal role model (nor mine). So consider for a moment: who do you look up to for inspiration on your own life map and practice vision?

Keep in mind that your team and your patients (who are the most important people in your office) care about two things:

1) **Confidence**. Do you personally, as the practice owner and visionary, have the confidence and care that they can see and feel in your office culture?

2) **Results**. Don't confuse "activity with proactivity." To win in sports, it's not about how long the game goes; it's about how you control it. If it takes less time, even better. Your patients don't want a longer procedure and will never complain when it takes less time. The sooner you are out of their mouth, the better, in their mind, assuming you are following the highest ethical standards in the way you treat and provide care.

Move ahead of the masses by leading your people with focus, motivation and a clear vision. Bend, but don't break. Work with your team and lead by example. When your team members are struggling, be there as a resource, but also let them learn. We like the saying "review but don't do" in my practice. I'm not sure who originally said it, but it's sound advice. You should review your systems and protocols with your team members, but don't do the work for them, for two reasons:

1. You don't have the time. Remember your ROT (return on time) is finite, so you must stick with spending yours on what's most important *today*.

2. No one learns when someone else does all of the talking or all of the work for them. Let your team members "skin their knees" (not literally), and they'll learn better and faster and more fully appreciate what you

have given them and have put into building a great practice. This is how you maximize ROP (return on people).

Like training for a race, you should help coach your employees and help them start the "marathon" of work that goes into running a growing dental practice. You should also be there to congratulate them and motivate them to finish the race. However, it is critical that you don't run the race for them or you won't be productive in your own work. The bulk of the race they need to do on their own, with you there as a solid "bookend" on either end of the journey. The top salespeople and sales trainers in the world use scripting to say the same message over and over--not in a badgering or political way, but rather to reaffirm your core values and practice vision. This will also make your best team members even better and weed out team members who are not a good fit for your team.

Dentaltown reported that many practice owners do not feel that their team members see the big picture and have a real vision of the practice. That is one of, if not your most important, roles as a practice owner. The survey stated that 53 percent of owners said the team understood their vision and carried it out (barely half); 43 percent said some do, but most are just there to collect a paycheck; and 4 percent felt like their team was not at all in line with their practice goals. We owe it to our teams and our patients to have a winning culture, where team members feel safe to share their ideas, and are constantly motivated and stretched to become all that they are capable of becoming.

Now that you've opened your mind more fully to your #1 asset - people - we will move into the next "P." Remember to always be developing your people with weekly meetings, daily training, goals and incentives, and positive feedback systems. Next, we'll move on to Pillar #4, which is about the Production and Productivity of your office. You'll learn about scheduling and efficiency as well as some of the systems you need to be really successful.

Chapter 7 Summary:

- Build meaningful relationships with four types of people: your team members, your patients, your vendors, and your community leaders.

- Do not accept complacency from your team members, and quickly release toxic team members. You cannot afford "indigestion" in your practice.

- People are like cars, they quickly get out of alignment. Invest in team member development and watch your practice grow.

- Most problems can be prevented or solved with great communication.

- Sight and sound (not the actual words spoken) account for 93% of communication.

- Use the 2/1 Rule of communication for follow up and for team member development. This will result with fewer remakes of lab work, fewer patients being upset, few team member issues, and most importantly - your growth numbers will take off.

- It's okay to fail. In fact, the most successful people do it often, and use it to to their advantage to learn from. Teach your team members to do the same.

Chapter Bonus: if you'd like a sample of my annual Leadership Planner, visit yourpracticegrowthbonuses.com for a free template.

Pillar #4: Are You Productive or Just Busy?

- Chapter Eight -

In this chapter, we'll dive further into opening up and developing your ROT (return on time), because simply seeing more and more patients won't make you more productive. You need to schedule and plan for a productive day, not just show up to the office and "see what happens." I do not believe in random luck.

Benjamin Franklin was quoted as saying, "I am a strong believer in luck and I find the harder I work, the more I have of it." He was also quoted as saying "diligence is the mother of good luck." Productivity in your office is only measured in results, which come only through systems and an office culture promoting **concentrated focus and diligent, hard work**. I once had a professor in my denture lab during dental school say, "Don't confuse effort with results." Your patients are only paying for one thing: RESULTS. Ensure your team understands that this is the only true measure of success in your practice. Some examples of ROT for you to measure are:

How many people did you help smile today?

How many patients left happier than when they arrived at your office?

How many days each week do you start and end with an on-time team huddle (the absolutely most important time of your patient production days)?

How many days each week do your team members start and leave on time (efficiency)?

Speed attracts money

According to the *Wall Street Journal*, in February 1852, "...a locomotive of the Michigan Southern railroad puffed into Chicago, connecting the breadbasket of the world directly with the Eastern U.S. for the first time. Instead of more than two weeks by horse, coach and canal boat, it would take just two days by rail to travel from New York City to Chicago. Goods, money and people were able to flow between the two booming cities faster than anyone had ever imagined." This was one of the big technologies of the Industrial Era that would forever change communication, travel and manufacturing. As technology speeds up today, so do the expectations of your patients. You have to be quick to implement valuable new systems into your practice and master them quickly to attract more out-of-pocket dollars from your patients. You have to **give them more than they are paying for** to be successful.

Since the Great Recession of 2008, the average income for U.S. dentists has been flat or declining. To be clear, even if your income is flat, it is actually declining. In January 2020, the *Wall Street Journal* reported the average income in the U.S. has risen by 0.4 percent and spending has increased by 0.2 percent. Multiplied by billions, that is a lot of green. Inflation inches up on us every year. I'm sure your staff are eager to get a pay increase or a bonus. Supplies and lab fees keep going up. You need to be constantly moving your production "thermometer" as we call it higher each month.

> *"When your desires are strong enough, you will appear to possess superhuman powers to achieve."*
>
> –Napoleon Hill

UNDERPRICED MASSAGES AREN'T SUSTAINABLE

One Friday night, my wife invited me on a date for a "Chinese Foot Massage" at a hidden office tucked away in a little shop in a strip mall a few miles away from my home.

This place sounds a little strange, right?

Well, it gets even better from here. This "Foot Massage" is actually a full body massage. You walk in, and they ask you one question--if you want feet only or full body. From there, no more questions or talking occurs; they just take over while you relax.

I used to think a professional massage was the weirdest thing until I tried it. I'm not sure how my wife ever found this place, but I think it was recommended to her. It's not your typical massage therapist style either. They use Chinese Reflexology, which is a little different, but very effective.

There are no frills here. They use old towels to keep you warm, and your feet are placed into a plastic bucket with a plastic liner and warm water. There are old massage-type chairs that look like recliners but have a hole in the headrest for when you lay face down.

Some traditional Chinese music plays from a little speaker in the room--there's no centralized sound system here. It's very clean and they are quite professional. As many "mom n' pop" shops go, they charge you a credit card fee, but it's cheap.

Really cheap.

The price was originally quoted at $45/hour, but they ran a special for $35/hour awhile back when my wife first went with some friends. Now, the sign on their door has a slash through $45/hour and it says $35/hour all of the time.

While they are fairly busy, I instantly wondered, "Are they actually making any money here?" It can't be free to hire licensed professionals. If my hygiene department ran that lean, we wouldn't make any money, but maybe these professionals have figured out a way to make it work with bare bones overhead. But my gut says they haven't. (Which is also why I gave them a big tip, because I feel for them and they did an excellent job.)

It appears to be a family-run business, with the owners and their children doing most of the work. It looks like they work long days and late hours, which is respectable, but probably not sustainable or a real "business" that can be sold. It's more of a self-employed job.

What fees are you slashing?
In which areas of service are you cutting back?
Are you adding up or removing the value you give to your patients?

I'm a much bigger fan of valuing up rather than discounting down. There will always be someone else lowering their fees or "rolling back" prices. You can play the low game or the high game, but usually if you are in the middle, you'll get burned.

Find ways to add value to your patient experience. Even a free bite adjustment on a crown or implant is added value. You're going to do it for free, anyway, if your patient needs it, so you might as well use it as a case acceptance tool or as part of your "selling proposition." Here are four ways this can go:

1. If your crown fee is $1000 and you have a 30 percent profit margin/70 percent overhead, and you "slash" your crown fee to try to gain more business, remember that you now have 82 percent overhead and a 18 percent profit margin.

2. Instead, find ways to value up, such as offering your patients more convenient appointment times (our evening and Saturday spots have filled up quickly since we started offering them about seven years ago).

3. Offer several options, with the higher priced one being an upgrade of better material, longer warranty, etc.

4. Always know your math. You can solve just about any problem in the world with the right math (that is why I was an economics major in college and why I love algebra - nerd, right?).

One of my favorite sayings on productivity comes from master marketer Dan Kennedy, who defines productivity as:

> ***Productivity is the deliberate, strategic investment***
>
> ***of your time, talent, intelligence, energy, resources,***
>
> ***opportunities in a manner calculated to move***
>
> ***you measurably closer to meaningful goals.***

Productivity is one of the most talked-about areas of your practice by most marketing companies and consultants. Yet most people who give you advice aren't truly productive in their own lives, and therefore are not ideal people to follow.

It is interesting to see how many different ways businesses can define productivity and what makes a productive workplace. In the dental office, it's clear that production is key to a growing and successful practice. If you have a hygiene team, you want to track and run that as a separate production team but also have great cross coordination. Doctor production and hygiene production are so integrated that if you set your schedule right and your goals correctly, the two will feed each other very well. It's a great way for doctors and hygienists to endorse each other and help patients receive a comprehensive treatment period.

It is absolutely key that you have a morning huddle, which is a mini meeting, for 10 to 15 minutes prior to seeing your first patient. Even if your schedule is wide open, make a plan and stick to it. Identify opportunities for your team and discuss how to increase your daily production. Make a fun game or offer rewards to the team when you hit your goal.

For best practices, I suggest you also have a "dehuddle" at the end of each production day. During the "dehuddle," you all get together and recap the day, stressing these important points: we time block certain areas of our day just to do large production procedures, and block off other areas of the day for less productive procedures. We define this as "sand," based on the Rock - Pebbles - Sand theory popularized by Stephen R. Covey in the 1990s. We also have two or three "rock boxes" each day which are exclusively limited to higher production procedures. Remember, the more you are producing, the more life-changing and health-giving dentistry you are providing for your patients, for whom you are ethically responsible to treat..

I also hold an "L-M" meeting with my treatment coordinator each day. L-M stands for Leader-Manager. Assuming you are the leader of your practice, you also need someone to manage the people and numbers, with you managing this person. This allows you to stay focused on the biggest opportunities, and allows you to train someone who can do many things better than you can in the way of practice management. Don't forget to keep to the numbers and results. This L-M meeting is a quick review of our daily goals, as well as any critical matters that arise. To learn how we run this effective meeting, set up a 30-minute practice assessment with my team at yourpracticegrowthbonuses.com.

We limit the number of "sand" appointments on our schedule each day, no matter what period. It is tempting to try to fit in more "sand," such as seeding crowns, bite adjustments, suture removals, etc., but they will quickly clog up your schedule and limit the amount of time that you will have for new or same-day dentistry. We use a template we call our "Gold Scheduling Guide." Even if your day looks kind of slow,, decide how many "sand" appointments you will allow in advance, and stick to this number so that you don't overfill your schedule. If you'd like a visual reminder of this, search online for Covey's video on rocks, pebbles and sand and share this great visualization with your team.

We have our practice management software set to ten-minute scheduling increments. We have a gold scheduling guide that defines how long each procedure takes, including one to two extra units, which allows 10 to 20 minutes for patients with lots of anxiety or other special needs. We then set a daily gap goal in each morning huddle, in which the assisting team and the hygiene team determines how far above or below our production is estimated to be to reach our daily net production goal.

Ensure that your treatment coordinator calculates net production on your schedule, not gross production. This allows you to calculate adjustments and also identifies potential areas of opportunity for new treatment. It's amazing how, on some days, 50 percent or more of our production comes from same-day treatment on the doctor and hygiene side. It becomes critical to block off these high production times so that team members don't accidentally fill them up with low production procedures.

We run surveys online, as well as on the postcards our patients complete. This helps us to gather data on their ideal times of the day. We then offer those times to our best patients first, including those who are on our in-house plan, and that helps us to determine the best high production times. You must balance convenience and accessibility for both new and existing patients, and at the same time, not crowd your schedule during those times. Crowding your schedule will bog down your team, make you run late and decrease your production. It's amazing how productivity and energy increase inversely to each other. When you're more productive, it forces you to be more organized, so that you put more effort into creating an efficient schedule. That's not to say that you must have everything figured out perfectly, but you should be at least 70 to 80 percent sure of what needs to happen within your schedule.

Track your production results on a daily, weekly, monthly, quarterly, and annual basis, but also check in halfway through each day. As Clayton Christiansen, the late Harvard professor, would say, you want to track leading indicators to see what's on the calendar. When you meet with your team each week, be sure to discuss this as you set your weekly goals by looking at the schedule ahead and what needs to be done to fill in the gaps to make your week great. We use a single gap, double gap, and triple gap measurement each day, and there are tiered bonuses and rewards for the team. One thing we like to do is have wooden coins in a fishbowl with different dollar amounts on them that team members draw from when we hit the gap. For example, a single gap is one coin. Double gap is two coins and triple gap is three coins. Those are a lot of fun to give to the team and everyone gets excited about it and creates a great sense of teamwork to get the job done well.

Do you have free "phubb" opportunities lying around in your practice?

When your team members call patients or accept an incoming call to take a payment or have a question answered, do you capitalize on that call? Returning calls, taking notes and maintaining your call-back list is a huge and very important task, but it is very time-consuming for your team members. To me, this is one of the most critical roles of your practice that builds trust with your patients and dramatically, yet indirectly, affects your practice growth and income.

Make sure your team members are familiar with the rule I call "PHUBB" Have them write it on a 3 x 5 card and keep it near your office phones as a reminder on how to capitalize on each call from an existing patient (or new patient, for that matter):

P - Profile updates (address, phone number, email)

H - Hygiene (recare appointment, periodontal treatment, or root canal/ortho/other specialty procedure follow-up)

U - Urgent or important treatment schedules and discussed (disease related examples: deep decay, tooth extraction, implants, ortho, root canals, etc.)

B - Billing up-to-date (outstanding balances paid)

B - Benefits (Insurance, payment plans, warranty on your work, special offers, in-house membership benefits)

If you'd like more training on how to use PHUBB to improve the phone skills of your team, give us a call at (801) 512-2987, or visit yourpracticegrowthbonuses.com.

When to refer: the four horsemen

You should never feel that you have to accept and treat every patient in your practice. Part of being a provider is not only providing the best dental care, but also providing the best personal care. When you are not a good match, or if you feel you cannot live up to expectations, now is a great time for your patient to go to a local dental school specialist. Here are my four horsemen for retaining or referring patients-- if your patient meets one* or more of the following criteria, you should likely refer. If they meet two or more criteria, you should most definitely refer:

1. They break appointments or never get any needed work done (*don't judge rashly; many patients may be fearful or scared or lack trust with dentists. This may take a year or more to help them overcome).

2. They complain about all dentists they've seen before as the problem for their teeth, not taking any personal responsibility.

3. They present an esthetic nightmare (patients who will be nearly impossible to please with outcome or appearance).

4. People who make late payments or break payment plan arrangements more than once.

You'll want to ensure you role play these scenarios with your team and practice daily. This simple exercise will not only save you thousands of dollars and hours of wasted time per year, but I'm confident that I can accelerate your rate of collections and scheduling appointments by 10 to 25 percent each year. When you call your credit card company or internet service provider, there is a reason that they confirm your address and contact information each time. As mentioned earlier in the book, the gold mine is in your existing list. These large companies have clearly done the research to prove it, or they wouldn't continue to verify who you are every time you call.

Now that we've discussed the Production Pillar, I hope that you are ready to implement these concepts right away. Set up a meeting with your key team members immediately and get these concepts working for you. If you don't take action, this book will simply be interesting to you. Don't dabble in interesting; that will never give you great results. Take action today. Next, we'll jump into Pillar #5, which is the Place you practice every day. Once you have these down, you'll be a master of the "3 Ps" for your practice.

Schedule to maximize your efficiency and profit

Over the years, we have developed an outline we call the "Gold Scheduling Guide." It is the legend for all team members to use when scheduling any procedure or exam type we offer. When a team member occasionally asks me,

"How long should I schedule this <crown, implant, etc.> for?" I ask them, "What does the Gold Scheduling Guide say?"

The reason I do this is because I'll mess it up if I'm not looking at this excellent guide. It is our legend for everything from delivering a denture to when we need to see a patient back for a new prescription vs calling it in over the phone, etc. It also helps us schedule what we call "gold" columns for our best and most productive patients, and "silver" columns for our less reliable or unconfirmed patients. If someone moves to "bronze" level, we dismiss them as a patient for too many cancelled or no-show visits. You can't tolerate that, or you'll always run late and lose on productivity. This is the 80/20 rule in action!

Hygiene scheduling strings

No-shows are an absolute killer, especially in your hygiene columns, because it's more difficult to get same-day or emergency treatment to patch up the holes on the hygiene side of your schedule. We developed something we call the "String Theory," which means we overbook hygiene by about 25 percent per day, then adjust each hour up or down 10 to 20 minutes to compensate for this.

It's like making a string into an "S" shape to represent your staggered schedule. Then you simply straighten it out and shorten it as your day goes on, to finish on time and hit the daily goal. Part of this concept is ratcheting down on your calls and electronic confirmation process, but some missed appointments are inevitable. **You absolutely cannot afford to let it ruin your daily goals!**

By using this strategy, you could have several no-shows on the same day and still beat your daily goal! Let me know how it works for you.

This chapter has focused on how to increase your production. Productivity must be both efficient and effective to provide A+ service to your patients while growing your practice and doing it on time regularly. In the next chapter we'll focus on your physical environment at the office.

Chapter 8 Summary:

- Being busy without being productive is expensive and time consuming.

- For every hour you spend on building systems in your office that make you productive, you will leverage 2 to 10 hours in the future by saving wasted time.

- Have a formula to avoid underpricing your services, or you will struggle to breakthrough to the next level.

- P.H.U.B.B. will multiply the effectiveness of your daily patient phone calls.

- The four horsemen tell you when to refer a patient out, in order to preserve the integrity of your practice and protect the experience of your best patients.

- Create an efficient schedule that works for your team. Not a schedule that your team has to constantly work for.

- If you do not take charge of your schedule, your patients will take charge of it for you and you will lack consistency in your production.

Pillar #5: Creating An Office That Works for You

- Chapter Nine -

When you think about it, you may spend more time in your office many days of the week than you do in your own home. Your team members will often do the same. So it is important that your office is not only clean, warm and inviting, but that it is a place that is conducive to high productivity and high case acceptance of treatments that your patients want. In this chapter we'll talk about making your practice not just a great place for dental treatment, but a "second home" for you and your team. If you want to make your practice a better and more productive place to be, then this chapter is for you!

A "Place" strategy is absolutely key to making your practice a great home for your team members and your patients. A clean and comfortable office can be one of your greatest marketing assets, especially when coupled with great visibility and signage outside.

In the smaller building in which I practiced for seven years, we didn't have access to or the ability to invest in a nice, big street sign. So instead, we bought these dumb little 24 x 36 inch stick-in-the-grass yard signs and ran different promotions and sayings on them. They were one of the highest ROI marketing assets we had for years. Don't let lack of funding or ordinances slow down your practice growth. Most of the time it's not funding or people we lack. It's lack of creativity that stifles your growth.

You'll need to budget into your weekly expenses an amount for repairs and maintenance. We have a large purchase account that we set up in our weekly transfer system that covers major upgrades of equipment. Small repairs can be covered with your SupplyX (supply expenses) budget. Just like an oil change on your vehicle or preventive dental maintenance for your patients, regular repairs from your weekly or monthly team member checklist will save you thousands of dollars of expenses. Additionally, it may potentially save you tens of thousands of dollars of production that could be lost on downtime from needed or deferred maintenance.

Have you ever heard the phrase, "location, location, location"? The location of your building is one of the most important elements of free marketing you'll ever find. My first location was on a very busy road, but the building was outdated and it was difficult for prospects to know what kind of business we were even running in it. Then we decided to put a big banner on the side of the building. All of a sudden, we began to attract more notice. Funny thing is, I knew very little about marketing at that point, so the sign wasn't even very good. It simply said, "Accepting new patients."

What a simple phrase we put on our sign! But it worked like magic to attract some great patients in need of care!

"Accepting new patients" does not sound exciting. It violates one of the most timeless marketing rules, which is to never be boring. It made no offer. It had no call to action. It showed nothing that set us apart. It was just a banner. But it showed that even something little like this could work. Imagine what kind of results you could get from a great sign! . I later found a new location in an existing building on a less busy road. Even though the building was nicer, we didn't get as much drive-by traffic. So we made these funny little grass yard signs and put different offers and headlines on them. Those little signs generated way more production than that one big sign on a busy street in our old location had produced. Imagine if we would have had this knowledge back then--how much better we could have done. We had no regrets, as it's all part of the learning process.

You should perform a monthly site assessment of your facility. My treatment coordinator or office manager does this. It's a simple one-page checklist where she walks around the inside and outside of the building and notes what looks great and what needs improvement. I'm amazed at how much trash you will find around your facility, or little things that need to be repaired that can really impact how your patients see you. An important part of this is your signage and your visibility. If you don't have a good outdoor sign, you need to think about investing in one. They are very expensive, but they will pay great dividends. The best part is, you can control the media on a sign. Google, Facebook or radio can change at any time, because the owners of those companies control the media. With your internal patient emails, your outdoor street signs, and the media types you use for marketing, however, you are in control. This means that they are valuable assets to your practice.

To obtain a free copy of our monthly "Good Vibes Site Assessment," visit the free bonuses and downloads page at: yourpracticegrowthbonuses.com.

Watch out for ocean stingrays

What is "stinging" the continued growth of your practice? We all have things that pop up, and as soon as you put that fire out, another will pop up. Just accept it as a fact of life and make a plan for the future. Early in 2020, I took my family on vacation to Puerto Vallarta, Mexico. It was my surprise Christmas gift to my wife and kids. If you haven't been to Puerto Vallarta, I highly recommend it. We went the all-inclusive route, and had everything we needed for a great time. Plus it's less than a four-hour direct flight from Salt Lake City.

We did leave the resorts a few times to take some Uber rides to visit downtown. We stopped at Walmart (which was a new experience for us - did you know that they sell motorcycles and stoves at Walmarts in Mexico?). The following day, we took a water taxi and went on a waterfall hike in Quimito (highly recommend) where we also found some awesome street tacos - just remember to bring pesos as ATM machines are hard to find. Off-site excursions are a lot of fun if you like to explore - but certainly are not needed in order to enjoy the experience. My kids had all of the beach time, boogie boarding, pool time, catamaran rides, arcade and foosball games, shuffleboard, virgin drinks at the juice bar, and nighttime shows they could handle. Plus the reserved restaurants had some fantastic fish tacos and chile relleno.

I don't think the trip could have gone much better. There were some pretty funny moments that you will experience on a trip that are unexpected but memorable. For me, this happened when I shut our resort beach rental booth down for a day with the "purple flag" from receiving my first (and hopefully only) stingray sting.

The beach rental company outside of our hotel had four flag colors posted each day. Green=safe water, yellow=use caution with larger waves, red=not safe to be in the water, and purple=dangerous marine wildlife/not safe to be in the water. We mostly had yellow conditions during our stay, which worked just fine, and only a few hours of red flag warnings one day. But on our last day, three of the five of us were boogie boarding, when suddenly I felt two quick, sharp "bites" on my right ankle, one just over the bone and one near my Achilles' tendon. It was so quick and intense, like a nail was pushed through my foot. I scooted across the next wave so fast I was back to shore in seconds - definitely beating my wife's speed on that ride.

When I sat down to observe what had just happened, I thought maybe something bit me because I was struck in two areas. It appeared that the stinger first tried to hit me in the ankle bone, but when it couldn't get through, it punctured me on the softer part of my foot instead. I had a three-inch welt and minor bleeding, and my foot began to feel numb, as it does when you sit on your leg funny and it "falls asleep."

Ouch!

After some reading up on it later that day, I discovered that stingrays are not aggressive toward humans, and only sting you to defend themselves if you step on one. Typically they swim in families and park in the sand during afternoon hours. (Hence the purple flag. When word got around in the resort that I was stung, they put that warning flag up because there were likely many more stingrays out. I was the one to whom people kept saying, "So, you're the guy we heard about that was stung.") I later learned that the "Stingray Shuffle" is the trick that surfers do as they scoot their feet along the sand to create movement. This warns stingrays that someone is coming and they swim away to avoid danger. Now I'll be dragging my feet more often!

What was I *really* afraid of?

I wasn't afraid of the pain or the bruise, but being a rookie, I wanted to ensure that I wouldn't have an allergic reaction or infection. So I asked a resort employee to take a look at my injury, and they immediately said, "stingray." I was quickly escorted to the on-site clinic. The doctor was very friendly, with a warm smile and laugh. He took me right into his examining room, where, before I knew it, I was being prepped for injections and given a bunch of pills I did not recognize. Through his broken English, I understood I would receive some localized numbing, followed by a cortisone shot so that the tingling in my foot didn't radiate higher. Then he applied some steroid and antibiotic cream and a bandage. The unmarked pills he gave me were painkillers and antihistamines (Claritin). I skipped taking the painkillers because I prefer Tylenol + ibuprofen over the counter but took the Claritin. Then I went over to the ATM (walking great!) and grabbed some cash to pay for the service.

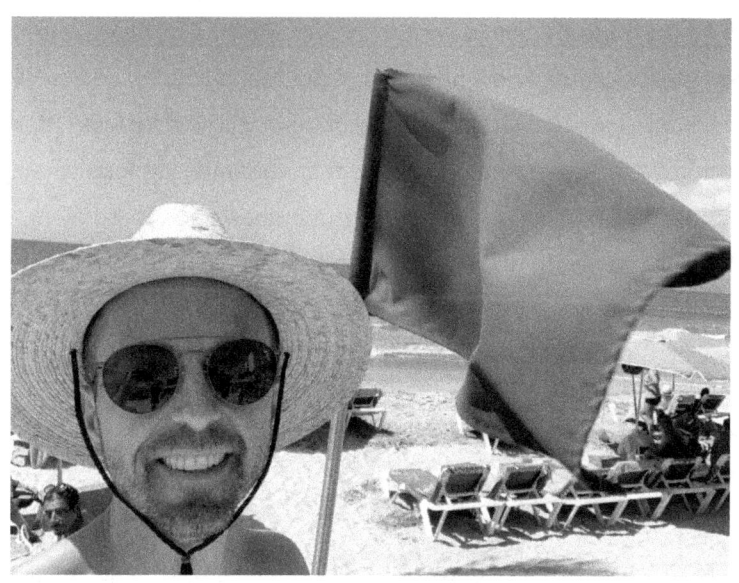

The purple flag

Within a couple of hours, the discomfort was 90 percent relieved, and I was happy to know that I could resume beach activities. I was very grateful for the experience, because it could have been much worse! NPR reported in 2014 that on Seal Beach in California, nearly 16,000 stingrays dwell in the water, but only about 400 stings are reported each year. Most people heal just fine afterward. Of course there are the fluke happenings, like when our favorite Crocodile Hunter, Steve Irwin, was stung in the chest, and it penetrated his heart and took his life back in 2006. That was a sad day for our family. We used to love watching his passion for animals and wildlife.

What kinds of "stings" terrify you in your practice? Do you stay up at night worrying about payroll, employees leaving, or where your new patient sources will come from? It would be easy for me to quit and never go back into the ocean again. Statistically it will probably never happen to me again. But most importantly, *I can't let one sting keep me from enjoying a vacation with my family. Even if I was stung again, I'd be better prepared and know what to do next.*

If you have anything that is "stinging" your practice or professional career right now, please let me know how I can help! Make your office the "place" you want to be for the long haul and a place your team will love to work. Start working today to improve the appearance, and more importantly, the functionality of your office. It doesn't have to be a Taj Mahal, but it does need to be clean, updated and highly functional. In the next chapter, we'll discuss how to boost the collections in your practice. Also visit yourpracticegrowthbonuses.com for a FREE copy of the monthly site assessment that you should have a team member use to analyze each month and report findings back to you.

Flow and functionality

My new office (which is in the late stages of final construction as I write this) was designed by one of the leanest and most efficient dental suppliers I have ever found. We used this model because it was designed by a dentist, for dentists. It maximizes our space, while keeping it functional and friendly for our team members and patients. If you'd like tips on renovating, an addition, or designing a new building, let me know. I'm happy to provide resources for you from people we know and trust from experience.

Now that you've made some notes on why your place of practice is so critical to your growth strategy, remember to keep it updated regularly. Your patients like to see that you are staying up-to-date, and especially making the dental environment fun with different prizes, contests and giveaways. Take the news and media off of your reception area TVs and radio, and update the environment to match your personality. Sit in every room in your practice and view it from the perspective of your patients. What do they see? That gives you free marketing tips for how to make it even better.

Chapter 9 Summary:

- *Simple and low cost internal marketing strategies will make your practice a significantly more profitable and more referralable place for your patients to visit.*

- *A clean, functional, convenient, and attractive office is a key marketing strategy.*

- *Have an assigned team member do a monthly "Good Vibes Site Assessment" of your practice.*

Pillar #6: Ouch! My Billing and Patient Accounts are Out of Control!

- Chapter Ten -

This chapter covers one of the most important Pillars in your practice: Collections. Money definitely isn't everything; you can always get it back, unlike your health or your time. But if you don't have money coming in, you can't pay your team, improve the "3 Ps," or reach your lifetime goals.

The collections growth formula

The way the office looks: from the street signs, to the restroom, to the drawers in the breakroom are one of our most important forms of marketing. Here is a collections growth formula that I came up with to boost your profits and velocity of increased money flowing into your practice:

$$(BTE + BPE + RS) \times MV = CG$$

Best team experience + Best patient experience + Repeatable systems

x Marketing Velocity = Collections Growth

Increasing your (revenue) collections is how you boost the payday for your team members as well as yourself. It's how you fund the new growth of your business. One day I was throwing out some ideas on a piece of sketch paper and I came up with this formula because I realized that the systems you have in your practice coupled with how quickly you get them implemented, repeated, and continually improved accelerates the growth of your practice.

In good times or bad, this formula will ensure that your practice stands the test of time. Remember it is a marathon, not a sprint, so you can't give up on anything. We aren't perfect and you don't need to be, either; you just need to remember to keep increasing thermometer goals for each of these to help push your team to the next level.

According to a 2020 article in the *Wall Street Journal*:

> *The average bear market wipes about 36% off the S&P 500 and lasts for about seven months, according to data compiled by Dow Jones Market Data.*

You have to be ready for these ups and downs in the economy during your years in practice. Just remember, practice ownership is a marathon, not a sprint. By making proper financial plans in your practice and weekly transfers into your "buckets," you'll be able to weather the storm. I am so grateful that, about a year prior to the 2020 Coronavirus Recession, I had become more aggressive in my weekly financial transfers in my practice. Although the government was making some small business grants available, I didn't want to get a loan to support my practice. If you get a loan when your numbers are down, you are double-dinged. Not only do you now have an additional monthly payment to make, but the income stream at the top of your funnel has already been throttled or shut off. With proper financial planning, you can push through these times and capitalize on the vast opportunities that arise when the dust settles. We actually had one of our best collections weeks of the year during the 2020 crisis, thanks to planning ahead of time.

Remember that your patients go through the same ups and downs you do during an economic cycle. You have to be sensitive to their needs and their lessened ability to pay their monthly payment plan bill or full copay during treatment. You need to plan ahead of time to address this without jeopardizing your accounts receivable or team incentives. You might even have to extend credit to those who may not be able to pay at all. Be sensitive to their needs and discuss how you will address this with your team in times of economic downturn. Be there for people and figure out a way to handle it that will be a win-win for everyone.

What investments are you making?

It is amazing how, as practice owners and small business owners, we can get distracted into making riskier types of investments with which we are less familiar. You must watch out for these distractions and be careful from whom you take advice. One guideline I suggest you establish is to be **careful of taking financial advice from people who make less money than you do**. It has nothing to do with arrogance or pride. If you wanted to be a top athlete, for example, think of who you would approach. If you wanted to become a professional tennis player, you wouldn't take lessons from an amateur. You would hire the best in the business.

At the same time, don't follow *everything* that successful businesses do. Larger companies are more bureaucratic and take longer to implement policies and marketing systems that can dramatically accelerate the growth of their business. The advantage you have as a practice owner is that you can turn the ship around quicker when you approach dangerous waters or when a big challenge arises. As a practice owner, you are preyed on by many types of salespeople who want your money and will try to hook you with ideas that will "make you more productive" or "boost your bottom line." Just be careful of shiny objects that come your way. A better approach is to map out your goals and plans for the month, quarter, and year, and then look for vendors and partners who can help you reach your goals. If it gets flipped the other way around, you could end up spending a lot of money on something that distracts you or causes you to invest in something that doesn't produce a positive return.

Although I have four businesses, the third and fourth ones piggyback on the first one, which is my practice. They are separate for legal and tax purposes, but I designed them to work harmoniously so that I don't get off course. Don't be one of the dentists who get caught up in speculative stock market investments or restaurants, or self-serve car washes, etc. First, invest more into your own dental practice, which can produce a much higher return on investment for you than mutual funds, real estate or retirement accounts.

I'm not suggesting you should not invest or have those things, but be sure to meet with your finance and tax advisor when you make a big decision. Most importantly, do the math before you make a decision. Remember this concept:

> *"If the math doesn't make sense, nothing else will."*

Keep in mind that your dental practice is the goose that lays the golden eggs, and your time, energy, and money spent there will likely produce the greatest return compared to any other investment over your lifetime.

Would you buy your practice again if you had to?

I was a terrible swimmer when I was younger, so much so that my wife laughed at me when we swam laps at the rec center when we were first married. After a little more instruction, I'm a bit better at it now. Mainly it was my breathing technique that I did not have down well and it slowed me down a lot. Other than playing in the pool as a kid, I didn't swim much, other than getting the merit badge in Boy Scouts. My wife is naturally a great swimmer, so it took me some practice to keep up with her.

You can't tread water and move ahead while conserving energy. So don't spread yourself too thin. Instead, focus on what you really want and make it your primary focus. Treading water actually consumes more of your energy and it moves you very slowly to the other end of the pool. The best use of your energy is to focus on:

1. Delivering high-production dentistry.
2. Planning growth strategies for your practice.
3. Training your top team members in management and leadership.

This has been Warren Buffett's winning formula in Berkshire Hathaway for many years and it's made him one of the wealthiest men on earth. You may not care to have as much money as he does, but his example teaches a valuable lesson. **He sticks with what he knows and what works for him, and he doesn't get caught up in shiny side projects or distractions.**

This may sound offensive, but if you hate owning or running your practice, then you should consider working for someone else. I mean it. If you'd rather just do dentistry, then find a way to do that and leave the management and marketing to someone better suited for it, or join a coaching group (shameless plug for our practice growth group) to help you put the right people in the right places. I was lecturing at an implant seminar some time back, and one of the dentists attending was complaining about the corporation that bought his practice and for which he now works. But you could see how happy he was focusing on implants and not running the practice, so it seems that he made the right decision.

How do you help your patients pay for treatment?

Credit card debt in the U.S. rose to a record $930 billion in recent years. According to the *Wall Street Journal*, "Americans spent aggressively in the final quarter of 2019 amid a strong economy and job market, and the proportion of people seriously behind on their payments increased." This was BEFORE the Coronavirus crisis of 2020, when the economy was very strong. So you can imagine how a credit crunch will impact your practice in this and future downturns.

Part of our "Bien 10" areas we track on our weekly scorecard include collections and accounts receivable. Although they are tightly intertwined, they are not the same thing. Before I paid enough attention to it, we would focus daily on collections, but often neglect the accounts receivable. This was a huge mistake, and I'm sharing this so that you can avoid it.

There are two major accounts receivable you need to measure:

1. Future Production-Collections % (ratio of your net production last month/ current accounts receivable without credits)
2. Healthy AR % (ratio of your good accounts receivable/total accounts receivable)

I cannot stress how important and critical it is to measure these on a weekly basis. Many "consultants" will tell you to measure 30+, 60+, 90+ days etc. But if you just narrow it down to these 2 indicators, you will have a rock-solid, secure, and well-oiled AR machine.

AR MEASUREMENT #1: FUTURE PRODUCTION-COLLECTIONS %

Calculate the total amount you had in net production last month (production - adjustments), then divide it by your total accounts receivable (without credits), and now you have your first critical AR number.

Like this:

Net production last month / Total AR without credits = Health AR %

Depending on your payment plan structure and flexibility, you should be around a 97 to 103 percent ratio for a good future forecast on your production. If your number is low, that means you are producing (doing) a lot of dentistry, but you are collecting far too little of it, and giving away many of your services for free.

You cannot afford to do that. You must pay your team members on time every payroll cycle, and that only happens with a healthy AR.

If your number is higher than 103 percent, you may be a bit too strict on your payment arrangements. That's why we have a 97 - 103 percent range: for some wiggle room. Low means you are not collecting what you produce, too high means you are closing off opportunities for your patients to accept more dentistry. Always be careful about who you qualify and how you do it, or you can get into trouble fast. Also don't be too strict or your case acceptance will drop. We use a soft credit check service for prequalification of our patients. But you have to find a happy medium, a sweet spot of how and who you will lend to. Remember, that does not include third-party financing, such as Care Credit, because that is paid in full to you, and Care Credit handles the accounts receivable on their end.

AR MEASUREMENT #2: HEALTHY AR %

The second, critical AR number that you track is calculated like this:

Receivables under 30 days + receivables in payment plans that are in good standing (and over 30 days) / total AR without credits

= Your Healthy AR %

You should shoot for 97.5 percent, give or take, depending on your flexibility and internal financing options.

You have to be open to the concept that you will lose a couple percent of your accounts receivable written off as bad debt each year if you really want to grow and increase your case acceptance. You will get better and more refined each year you stick with it. Owning a dental practice is a marathon, not a sprint. If you keep this number tighter than 97.5 percent, that's okay, but your overall collections number will also remain smaller due to less treatment being accepted and rendered.

I've found that it's worth the slight risk to know that my case acceptance and total collections goes up dramatically by helping more people get the care they want sooner, avoiding root canals, etc. My treatment coordinator was shocked when I first started having her track this number. She quickly realized that our accounts receivable had started to get out of hand because we were essentially providing "free interest" for too many people who were not paying because we weren't getting their statements to them in a timely manner.

Your front office team should sound the alarm when an account goes beyond 30 days. Get your patient involved if necessary. In your new patient packet, provide a clause (under advice of your legal counsel) saying that insurance claims that go beyond 30 days are the responsibility of the patient. Help them understand this at every step of the way and keep them in the loop.

Studies have shown that past due balances over 90 days have about a three percent average collection rate. That means anyone who is 90 days past due on their payment, with the exception of people whose monthly payment plans are in good standing, have a very, very low chance of paying you. If you have $100,000 in AR over 90 days, for example, you're likely to <u>only collect $3,000</u> of it and <u>write off $97,000</u>. Do you really want to do that?

We do not send patients to collections as of a couple years ago, because we feel it is our fault for not managing the terms of their account, not theirs. We shouldn't have given financing to these people to begin with. Sending someone to collections is a lose-lose scenario and not good for anyone, in my opinion, as far as dental practice goes. If you sell cars or real estate, that's a different situation, because there is real property you can repossess. But you can't, nor would you want to, go and repossess the crown on your patient. You have to manage that properly upfront in order to set yourself up for success.

Manage AR from the start or refer them to a low-cost clinic. Otherwise, you're probably working for free, but still have the same bills to pay. Unfortunately, some people are seeking to take advantage of practice owners, but most people have good intentions. Life simply gets in the way sometimes, and there's always another unexpected expense or bill that pops up. So be prepared and have well-thought-out guidelines. If you'd like more tools and resources on this, visit yourpracticegrowthbonues.com for some additional tools, or contact my office.

Be a tortoise - be a long term winner

You've likely heard the old story of the tortoise and the hare. Essentially, the tortoise wins because he has the long-term, marathon mentality, while the hare is on a stop-go, unfocused, take-it-for granted run. Marketing legend Dan Kennedy says that people start quitting your business or lose interest the minute they start. Studies on the psychology of buying have found that as buyers, our interest is highest right when we purchase something. Then it immediately begins to drop. Sometimes that act of going to buy, or knowing what you are going to buy, generates more "feel-goodness" than does the actual product or service that you receive.

For example, if you're buying a new car, day one is the most exciting, and then it fades every day from there, until you feel one of these three ways about your purchase:

1) You begin to take it for granted

2) You get tired of it

3) You feel you need to buy a new one.

It's how I've often felt about Christmas - meaning that Christmas Eve is the MOST exciting day of the season for me, because of all the excitement and anticipation (and knowing the holiday rush will soon be over).

So you have to keep things interesting, new and exciting, constantly building the relationship to bring your patients back for their next visit. The day of their checkup or new implant is THE most exciting day for your patient. It's also the best time to help them accept more treatment and get them scheduled for their next visit, because the feel-good feelings are at their highest on that day.

How do you celebrate with your patients? How do you make it fun at your office?

This is why I believe most hygiene programs in our practices are underutilized. The perceived need of doctor treatment is higher: pain, broken teeth, bad breath, bleeding mouth, all of them feel more important to the average person, and therefore people will pay more and come in sooner to have these services done.

Where are the highest opportunity recurring collections (revenue) in your practice?

When it comes to prevention (a word that does not have any sizzle or excitement), people often put it off, even though, in fact, everyone DOES NEED a checkup and cleaning periodically. Think about it: do you get excited to go get an oil change on your car? Probably not, but you are likely excited to drive your car again after the transmission goes out or the engine fails. Hygiene is a huge source of recurring revenue, and with a trained hygienist and recare program, it is the closest thing to passive income (next to real estate if you own your building) that you can gain in your practice if you are a solo doctor.

Dropbox is an exemplary company that has done well with its recurring revenue program. Here's how *Investor's Business Daily* described it:

"Dropbox makes file-sharing software that enables collaboration among work teams. Users pay a monthly fee for larger storage space. Thus, converting free users to paid accounts is a key growth driver. Of more than 600 million users, only 14.3 million were paying customers at the end of 2019. That's up nearly 12% from 2018....One of the company's main metrics is total annual recurring revenue, which is the key indicator of the trajectory of its business

performance....It represents the amount of revenue Dropbox expects to recur, helps measure the progress of initiatives, and serves as an indicator of future growth. In the fourth quarter, total annual recurring revenue was $1.82 billion, up 3% from Q3 and about 20% from the year-ago period."

Dropbox is a great example of how to build a recurring collections stream in your practice. Offer something valuable for people to join (for them a free basic plan) and then focus on creating a lifetime customer (or patient) who pays you monthly/annually and continually gets great value in the product or service.

Other ways to build recurring revenue into your practice include hiring associates and well-trained assistants, and offering payment plans. Just ensure you have daily reports to track all of these metrics and hold the proper team members accountable to reporting back on them.

A great exercise this week is to break down your collections by the following:

- Hygiene collections by provider
- Doctor collections by provider
- Healthy AR % & Future P-C %, 90+ accounts receivable (90+ is what we call "bad AR" in the extreme danger zone, unless it's part of a current payment plan)
- Over-the-counter collections (non insurance/patient portions paid)
- Insurance collections

Average these out with six to 12 months of data, and you'll soon see where your revenue (collections) really come from. This will help you make better decisions on things such as adding more providers, offering more or fewer payment plans, accepting or dropping insurance plans, etc. In my office, I was pleasantly surprised years ago to see that nearly two-thirds of our payments come from patients, whether cash pay or copayment. For my practice philosophy, this means I'm not overly dependent on insurance, which wouldn't match our service model. Even though we are very insurance friendly in my practice, we don't believe in making decisions solely based on insurance. But my office and yours are different, and so will your recipe be for success. You just need to make sure you have the right ingredients to flourish.

Helping your team

I believe an important part of our role as practice owners is to help our team members develop professionally and personally. One way you can do this is to teach your team members sound financial advice. This comes through teaching them about debt elimination, money management and good stewardship. You have to show and teach them this every day by example and by letting them learn on their own. Don't expect anyone on your team to offer solid financial advice, but give them the opportunity to learn it. I would love if one day, everyone on my team was debt free outside of a home mortgage. You should work with your team and team leaders to check in on their personal goals as well periodically, and managing collections is a great tool to do this.

Thomas Stanley, author of *The Millionaire Next Door*, and his fascinating follow-up book, *The Millionaire Mind*, researched and developed 20 years of studies on how millionaires got to where they are today. Keep in mind these books were written back in the 1990s, but the principles still apply wholeheartedly today. Here are a few of his findings about millionaires:

- They **allocate their time, energy and money efficiently**, in ways conducive to building wealth.
- They believe that financial independence is **more important than displaying** high social status.
- Their **adult children are economically self-sufficient.**

- Prodigious accumulators of wealth spend **nearly twice as many hours per month planning their investments as under-accumulators of wealth**.

- Ninety percent of millionaires live in homes valued below $1 million; 28.3 percent live in homes valued at $300,000 or less.

- On average, millionaires have a **mortgage that is less than one-third of the value of their homes**.

- On average most millionaires **invest 20 percent of their income.**

- The majority of wealthy people are married and stay married to the same person.

Many doctors can take lessons from this research. I read this book shortly after dental school. It really made me reflect on what I measured as successful, and where I wanted to be in five, ten or 20 years. Think about it: do you want to *look* like a doctor, or do you want to look like someone who is truly successful? There is a difference. Stanley also found that after a certain point, income level had much less to do with how much someone makes in a year, but rather on what they do with it. This is not taught in dental school, or even most business schools, for that matter. In obtaining my economics degree in college, we talked and learned a lot about finance and banking, and I really value that learning experience. However, we learned very little about personal finance and managing it properly, and it still isn't taught in most business schools today. It comes from learning in the trenches and refining the art of good discipline and rational decision making.

The average American household spent (only) just under $29 on books in 2018, according to Statista.com. But the average household spends thousands on media and movies as well as mobile apps. This is both a telling and an alarming statistic. Worse yet, the average household spent $42 per year on books in 2012 and $52 per year in 2007. We are reading less!

We think we don't have time to read, yet we squander away thousands of hours a year on wasted time. Sure, we all have to have fun and let loose, but teach your team the importance of developing themselves, and most importantly, lead by example.

You can do much in developing yourself and developing your people through continuous learning and improvement. CE courses are great, but they are the minimum requirement. You should also spend dedicated and regular time developing yourself and your team in leadership, sound financial literacy, and personal development.

This ties into my philosophy that financial deposits are incredibly important, but relationship deposits into people, and the value you can create as a practice owner and a provider are even more valuable to the people in your sphere of influence.

Your combined lab and supply budget should be under 15 percent of your total adjusted collections. Teach your team why and how this works, and they will gain more respect for how the practice operates and how critical consistent collections and financial literacy are.

Practice profits bucket system

We don't have time to dig deep into this topic in this book, but it is covered in depth as part of our Practice Growth Monthly Membership Program (my shameless plug here...). With this system, you create multiple accounts, or "buckets," at your bank or credit union. You then transfer money from your income account each week to respective sub accounts to *really* see where your money is going. Accounts are great to have as part of your team, and are really good for maximizing your tax savings and strategizing. The problem is that your income statement and what is actually in your bank account are two totally different things.

I learned this years ago when I wondered why my tax professional said that I had made all of this money, but my account didn't reflect it. A big discrepancy! Where did all of that money go? It was because of this difference:

Marketing Money Math vs. Accountant Math

The former is what you should focus on to grow your practice, and leave the latter up to your tax professionals. Accountants provide great advice, and I really appreciate mine, but don't let them be the captain of your ship. **You have to take those reins.** I learned through trial, error, and great advice from mentors and successful business owners, and have never looked back with this program I adapted for growing dental practices. To learn more, call or visit our website.

How to fail before you start

Here are some common traits in practices that are a sure way to set yourself up for financial trouble, before you even start your day:

1. Not having flexible, written-out financial guidelines in place. Remember to be flexible, but don't break. Use terms such as, "We ask for a $200 initial investment to schedule the appointment," not, "Our policy is that you pay $200 before you schedule the appointment."

2. Not having daily written goals set for doctor production, hygiene production, collections and new patients. If you don't write these down and talk about them in your AM huddle, you are sure never to hit them.

3. Not keeping to a schedule. Start on time and finish on time, every day. Make exceptions for "rocks" (large treatment plans) or emergency treatment with 20 minutes or so of leniency added onto your finishing time at the end of the day. Go the extra mile for patients who have the most work to do or are in pain.

Now that we've covered collections and AR, you'll want to pay much closer attention to these numbers. A daily collection and production goal is a must in your morning huddles. Then ask your key team members HOW they plan to achieve them. You have a critical role in the production in your practice, and every team member should be accountable for a piece of that pie. In the next chapter, we'll conclude with making your practice an outstanding experience for your patients--one that goes well beyond teeth and dental care.

Chapter 10 Summary:

- *Implement the collections growth formula: best team experience + best patient experience + plus repeatable systems x by marketing velocity = collections growth.*

- *Investing directly in your practice is usually the best and highest return on investment for business owners.*

- *When the math in any practice decision doesn't make sense, nothing else will.*

- *Would you buy your practice again?*

- *Use the Healthy AR and Future P-C guidelines to track your accounts receivable and to minimize huge and costly write offs.*

- *Offer flexible but guided payment options for your patients.*

- *Use the Practice Profits Bucket System for weekly transfers, and most importantly to increase your profit account.*

Pillar #7: What Really Counts at the End of the Day

- Chapter Eleven -

By this point in the book, I hope you've made some notes on what you'll implement starting today. If you're like me, you'll want to go back to the areas you need to reread or that you feel will make the biggest impact on your practice, review them, and start writing down your goals for the quarter and year. Do the math and then work backwards to today to map out your plan. Then, take those principles and create strategies and smaller tactics to get there. It's easy to underestimate what you can actually accomplish in a quarter or year, so push yourself and your team to do great things.

In this final chapter, we'll conclude with the most important number to measure in your practice--the experience each patient feels in your office! This is tracked by all of the 7 Pillars and the size of the ROI on your RMAP. Keep in mind, your patients who have a great experience will do one to three of the following things:

1. Come to your office more frequently for dental care (higher frequency/recare).
2. Accept more comprehensive treatment plans (higher production).
3. Refer more (higher appreciation for who you are).

The experience inside your practice actually starts outside of your building. It happens when someone hears about you, then calls you or emails you, then you call them back to discuss their first visit in your office, then they step inside your door. The cycle repeats over and over as you retain and grow your patient base. The experience people have is the way you build trust, grow your referral program, and increase your collections, which benefits your team and supplies the continued growth of your practice.

We call these "Relationship Deposits," and they are the most important type of deposits you'll ever have in your career. How many lives did you change? How much trust did you build with your team and patients? How many smiles did you give? How many minds did you put at ease for fearful patients?

How do people feel inside of your four walls?

Have you ever realized that dental offices are scary places to many people? Drills, invading personal space (literally being in their faces), noises, shots, pulling teeth, root canals. The list goes on and on. Never take for granted that just because you are comfortable with dental science, many of your patients are not, and most could care less about the clinical side of dentistry. They care more about you, especially if they feel you care even more about them.

This goes beyond just the experience your patients have with you. Just as important, and in fact, even more important, is the experience your team members have as part of your office culture. You need to provide great leadership and be an example of how to do the right thing and maintain your core values in your practice. In the beginning of this book, you learned about supply versus demand in the marketplace. In order to keep a consistent supply of team members and great applicants coming your way, you need to meet and exceed the demands in the labor marketplace.

One of the biggest observations I had during the COVID-19 pandemic when one-third to two-thirds of practices were closed or had very limited open hours was the abandonment of patients. Even if you can't physically see your patients, you can still send them a newsletter, email, phone call or video teledentistry call. Essentially, much of our profession was saying, "Hey, since you can't come and pay me or give me your insurance benefits, I don't care about you right now."

You probably don't really think that way, but can't you see how your patients and team members could feel and perceive that as reality?

It's time to step up to the next level and really care for your team members and patients. If you don't, your office will have a revolving door, where you lose new patients (the most expensive type of patient) just as quick as you gain them. That is a very expensive and unsustainable model.

You will have to make tough decisions along the way, and so will your team managers. It's a critical part of what you do, and something that many practice owners do not like to face. You will have to dismiss certain team members and bad patients. But do it quickly and respectfully. Without making tough decisions, you will plateau and never go to the next level. If you're content where you are and you don't care about going to the next level, then that's just fine. But you have to be frank and honest with yourself on what goals you have laid out and where you want to be in the next one, five, and ten years from today. When in doubt, overdeliver on the value given to both your team members and your patients. However, be sure to establish and continually remind your team of the well-defined boundaries you've given them to be part of your cause. Give them freedom within those boundaries, but not the unwarranted ability to go outside of them.

Early on, I learned that if I have to decide between being a team member's "friend" and being their leader, the latter is the better option. This means that you should be very generous with the opportunities you provide your team members, but establish expectations of what they need to do to get there. Make your environment fun and a great place to work. One of our core values is to have fun and laugh every day. But that doesn't mean we goof around all the time or allow sloppy work or inefficient systems. It's actually the opposite. Because we have set such a high expectation and standard in my office, we laugh and have fun so that we don't take life too seriously outside of work. You need to find these boundaries with your team and put them in writing. You should also have an employee handbook (contact your payroll provider if you don't have one) containing these written boundaries, and refer to them often.

We post our core values on our quarterly planning sheets as well as in our break room and in our morning huddle outline. They are everywhere intentionally. When a team member is not doing their job correctly or they are neglecting responsibilities, I remind them of our core values and let them know how much I care that they do well and that I expect better of them. Use these as your disciplinary guidelines, not personal shots or subjective reasoning.

If you do this in a way that shows that you want to help them develop and grow, they will appreciate it and learn to take it as constructive feedback. In the book, *Traction*, Gino Wickman calls this "constructive conflict," and it is something you need to have in order to be open and honest with your team members. You must be open and honest with yourself as well and allow team members to provide you with feedback on their experience, their ideas and how they can contribute to your team. Sometimes the biggest growth will come from looking at yourself in the mirror and having the data on what you need to do to improve.

Take your team out to dinner

In January 2020, I took my dental practice team out for a New Year's Dinner at Valter's Osteria in downtown Salt Lake City. Valter's is not your typical Italian restaurant.

Valter, the founder and owner, walks around with his big head of white hair, finely dressed in a suit, and shares a smile and a strong Italian accented "hello" with his guests. His regulars get a warm hug at the door or at their table. These actions work well for him, as the nine of us ran up a bill of $800+ with tip in just a couple of hours.

My wife and I enjoy treating them to a dinner every New Year, and my team was very appreciative. They all loved their meals and, as always, my wife absolutely loved their bread.

Valter is full of personality, and that cannot be copied or replicated.

Are you fearful of changes coming your way in dentistry? Do you lie awake at night worrying about your team or what your patients will think of their experience in your practice? If so, you need a new or updated strategy for being *the place to go* for your patients. What makes you different?

If there's one thing no corporate practice or new office on the block can copy from you, it's your personality. Kennedy calls this "personality in copy" when referring to the way you communicate with your patients, which includes recare letters and appointment reminder emails that you send to them.

What makes you different? What personal experiences do you have to share? Why should a patient come see you versus all other available options, **including options that have nothing to do with a dentist?** Have you ever realized that vacations, new cars and shopping on Amazon.com are *your real competition*, not your colleague down the street?

You need to communicate your personality and the personality of your team like Valter does. You don't have to be exactly like him, but you need to be **you** and share your stories and personality like he does. You need to share your team members' stories, too (with their permission). It is your unique identifier and should be part of your USP (unique selling proposition) if it isn't already. Do you have smiling, trust and testimonial-building faces in your newsletter, **or just articles about teeth that will bore or even scare many of your patients?**

By sharing your personality on a daily, weekly and monthly basis with both your team and your patients, you will build lasting relationships that are unique. You will also dramatically increase the frequency with which your patients visit your office, which will help you reach the goals you have set this year. Then continue to share this message over and over.

If you are going to be in downtown Salt Lake City anytime soon, I suggest you make a reservation at Valter's in advance, as they get completely booked every weekend. I recommend the salmon and any of their pasta and bread. If you take your team, make sure you take some photos of it and share it with your patients in an email or newsletter. It is part of your RMAP - Relationship Marketing Action Plan.

Have some M&MS

My wife and I have a group of friends who get together once a month or so on a weekend for "Game Night." This often consists of mostly talking, socializing and eating treats, but it does involve different card or board games played as teams, either in couples or as men versus women. Megan usually outscores me, except for games on trivia or memory, which is my strong point.

Game Night is really about the social aspect and eating sweets together. Someone usually brings a big tub of peanut M&Ms, which are a crowd favorite. Although not my top pick, I have begun to enjoy them more over the years.

In growing your practice, there is an M&M formula on how you should spend your time and initiate a culture with the right attitude and team members. This formula is simple, but that doesn't mean it's always easy. However, it is vital for your success in reaching your desired destination, whether you want to be a single doctor practice, multi doctor practice, or sell your practice to a bigger group or corporation.

One half of your business and family life are dependent on the first "M" - Mindset. The other half of your business is dependent on the other "M" - Methods.

Let's break each one down.

Mindset is how you think about your day, both personally and professionally. It's how you view your world and the people around you. Most importantly, your mindset is how you act vs. react to situations, challenges and experiences all around you. I'm certainly not perfect, nor do I pretend to be. However, I know that things happen for a reason, and there's a lesson to be learned within every challenge. As a business owner and leader in your community, your job is to turn these situations, challenges and experiences into valuable opportunities and help others to do the same.

Mindset is your thinking, your daily routine, and your outlook on your practice's future. Without it, you are dead in the water. Without the right mindset, you'll change directions every year when the emotional challenges of practice ownership come your way. You may be influenced by insurance pressures, slashing your fees, or giving in to patients who do not fit your culture. You may give in to poorly managing team members or worse yet, not helping them reach their optimum potential. You have the power to provide the influence and growth mindset to take your practice to the next level, and to attract the right people to grow with you.

In the ESPN documentary *The Last Dance*, superstar Michael Jordan comes out of retirement from baseball after a major league players' strike and goes back into professional basketball. That season, his team fell short of beating the Orlando Magic in the NBA playoffs.

Most players would take some time off right after a devastating loss like that. What did Michael do? He was back in the gym the very next day, working harder than ever. His philosophy was, if someone was going to commit three hours to watching him play, he had an obligation to provide an outstanding performance for the fans, teammates and spectators.

He showed similar commitment several years before after getting beat up by the "Bad Boys" of the Detroit Pistons in the playoffs. He was so sick and tired of losing to them that he was in the gym hitting the weights and getting stronger. It paid off when the Bulls beat the Pistons the next season.

Jerry Rice was known to be at practice the next day after winning the Super Bowl. Both of these athletes show elite-level commitment. **How would that level of commitment launch your practice to the next level?**

There is a concept about mindset that has been described by renowned speaker and coach Lee Millteer, who was quoted as saying, "When you ask yourself a question, your brain - which is literally a computer - searches for resources and answers to that particular question." Use this to your advantage. Work proper exercise, rest and a good diet into your daily routine to keep that computer functioning properly. As described in the book, *Deep Work*, you do some of your best problem-solving when you aren't focused directly on those problems. The higher neuronal capacity of your unconscious mind goes to work.

Remember that the greatest assets in your practice are the people that you work with. This includes your relationship with vendors, team members, and patients. Great team members are your number one asset, and your patients are a close number two. Without great team members, you will have holes in your bucket and your system will not operate well enough to help you grow. Your team members are essentially a walking billboard for your practice. Do they promote you outside of work? Do they refer their friends and family to you? Do they see your office as an important part of their life or just as a job?

The sad truth is that if you aren't sure, that means your team probably isn't doing much to help you grow your practice. It's eye-opening to see what your team members say behind your back. Several times a year, ask your office manager to conduct a survey about your office. Share the highly rated areas of your practice with your team members, which further proves their morale and engagement in working for you.

Whether you have perfected them or not, the systems you have (or the systems that are broken in your office right now) are a mirror reflection of you personally and professionally. It's **your** name on the door. It's **your** culture that you build (or neglect to build) that is felt by your team and patients inside those four walls.

Methods are how you do things. Your methodology is how you build systems, plan your day, and get people around you who can help you stay organized and goal-driven. As you grow, you will constantly have to refine your methods and make them better. However, to paraphrase, as Adam Witty, owner of Advantage | ForbesBooks says, being successful is much more about implementation than it is invention. New, shiny objects will not make your practice better or your life easier, by themselves. You have to use them regularly, and learn to use them better, in order to excel. Often, you already have the tools in front of you, but you need to go out and build and repair the projects you already have under your nose.

Most New Year's Resolutions NEVER HAPPEN. We start with great intentions, but by week two, we are already waning in our commitments. If you recommit yourself each week to your practice and life goals, you'll be heads above the rest. Give systems, processes and previous ideas you've implemented a real chance to work. If your first implant or clear aligner case you ever started didn't work out as intended, would you quit? Of course not, but that's what most people do with their goals, and you don't want to be most people. Most people struggle through life financially, living in debt and paycheck to paycheck--even dentists and business owners. Move above the turmoil, and put the life you want in place today, with the right methods of success in front of you.

Strive for perfection, but don't expect it

"Practice makes perfect" isn't quite accurate. Otherwise, your dental procedures would be 100 percent successful, because you've practiced them a whole lot, whether in school or in your practice. Legendary coach Vince Lombardi said, ***"perfect practice makes perfect,"*** which is more accurate. You'll never have a perfect practice, but you don't need to for a high level of success. You just need to be really good. There is a military principle that says you only need 70 percent of the information to move ahead or make a decision to proceed. We typically use 80 percent, but you get the idea. In terms of grades, you only need a B to be good enough at something. I'm not suggesting you ever compromise your clinical care; always shoot for the moon. But in marketing, team building, or growing your practice, don't let "analysis paralysis" stop you from doing great things. Have most of the information or most of the outline done and then go for it! You can tweak and adjust as you go.

Strive for perfecting, but never hold yourself to being perfect. You should always aim for perfection as your gold standard, but don't beat yourself up when you don't get there. As a dentist, you probably have some level of perfectionist qualities in the way you look at your work. You must be your best, but don't expect to be perfect. To get an "A," you can still miss a couple of questions on a test. Make a "good enough" game plan and get started today. **What are you waiting for?**

Growing your practice is an ongoing challenge and can be a very fun opportunity. If you don't see growing your practice as an opportunity or a challenge you want to work on, you should seriously consider selling your practice or working for another office. All of the work that goes on behind the scenes and after hours that your patients and team do not see simply isn't worth it for the money alone. It's a great privilege to own a dental practice, but as you know, there's a lot of work involved. Practice ownership is really about creating a legacy for your patients and team and building a culture that's more than simply fixing teeth. You treat people first and teeth second, not the other way around. You can build a practice that is a resource for your community and also a great opportunity to teach your team members about valuable life lessons, personal finance, and leadership. I hope this book helps you take your practice to the next level on the continuous path of growth.

As dental professionals, we love predictable results. Do you want your root canals, composite bonding, or dental implants to be 90 to 99 percent successful? In marketing, some of the campaigns you run will have less than half of a percent response rate. That's when you might feel like giving up, because that seems like a very poor result. What you have to remember is the value of that half percent, which can be astronomical. You may send out 10,000 postcards and only get a few responses. If you send them to the right people, however, your message will not fall on deaf ears, and you will reach an audience that is eager and ready to accept your offered treatment. The magnitude of great systems and great marketing in your office does not have to be perfect, nor does it have to be for everybody, and, in fact, it shouldn't be. What you should focus on is doing more with the right people rather than trying to be everything to everybody, which really means you won't be anything to anybody.

For more resources, visit www.yourpracticegrowthbonuses.com or reach out to my office. We are happy to help. It's what we do, and what gets us excited is helping others maximize the valuable resources we have to offer.

New opportunities arising in practice leadership

Right now, as the dental landscape is becoming a crazy, shaken-up place, start **working on sharpening your mindset and your methods, which are exponentially more important than ever.** If you are busy with patients, use some of your downtime, early mornings (my preferred time) or holiday breaks as an opportunity to focus your clarity and vision, and re-evaluate your long-term goals. I promise you'll come out of these thought-provoking sessions with a stronger and clearer vision than ever.

I hope you enjoyed reading this book as much as I did putting it together. I had you in mind, a proactive owner, just like me, who is looking to grow the practice of your dreams, starting today. As new challenges arise, both inside your practice and in the outside economy, new opportunities are forming. Now that you have the tools to recognize them, *it's time to go out and put them to work.*

There is no "easy button"

Implement one small but powerful thing each month for the next year, and all of a sudden, you'll have 12 new things working for you, to boost your practice. Do three new things per month for a year, and you'll end up with 36 new and profitable changes working to your advantage, while simultaneously providing an enhanced experience for your patients and team members.

As practice owners, we often want to have a quick and easy fix. We just want to send a few postcards, get a new implant kit, buy CAD/CAM technology, get Invisialign certified, etc. to make our practices more productive. All of these are good things in the right situation, but alone, they are <u>NOT strategies to grow your practice</u>. They are tools to be used with the right growth strategy. In fact, when used incorrectly, they can cause a loss of revenue in the form of negative profit.

I've learned the hard way, and now I've found the easier way. I've learned that you must be improving multiple areas simultaneously in order to really make things work quickly, efficiently, and profitably. If you tell a few of your patients that you now offer implants, I promise droves of people won't come running to your office. Dental treatment just isn't that exciting to most people. But I can promise you that if you send out a consistent message, month after month, being persistent but not pushy, then you will gain some great new referrals and great complex and restorative cases over and over again. A one-time boost simply won't pay the bills in today's environment. Your system needs to be repeatable. This is the practice environment we are living in today.

I'll be candid. If you aren't willing to do these things, you must accept mediocrity, and the increasing costs of doing business with more downward pressure from outside forces. It's an uphill battle. Of course, no one is forcing you to do these things, but my job is to tell you what has worked for me and what hasn't worked, to benefit your future. If I'm not straight with you, then this book is nothing more than a "quick read." Instead, I want you to prosper from it, both financially and in your relationships with your team and community.

None of this is your fault or a result of your decisions. This is how we are programmed. This is how we were taught in dental school. But it's time to change from old school to new school.

If you change the experience in your practice to a place where people **want** to go, rather than where they **have** to go, then you can create a very valuable asset to you, your team, and your community. You can grow and thrive better than ever by putting together your RMAP (Relationship Marketing Action Plan) and then executing it on a monthly basis.

Classic author Napoleon Hill, who wrote as an advisor to President Roosevelt, studied billionaires, and wrote *Think and Grow Rich*, among other great titles, once stated:

> *"Every adversity, every failure, every heartbreak, carries with it the seed of an equal or greater benefit."*

Now, go out and do it!

Only **you** have the power to put your practice on track to reach your life goals and help your team reach theirs. Regardless of your situation, there's no time like the present to make this happen. In this book, we've covered the 7 Pillars of Growth Strategies based on over a decade of real-world practice ownership experience. Now, go back through and use this book as a reference as you implement or restore each pillar in your practice.

Psychologists have taught us that we only retain about 50 percent of what we learn for 48 hours. This is why I dog-ear, highlight and mark up the best books I own to reread them and use them as a textbook for success. If you feel this book can help you, then do the same with it. Of course, if you have questions, visit our website and we'll be glad to help you.

After a couple of weeks, you will have forgotten almost everything you've learned here and in other books, unless you reread it or refresh yourself on the information. Life gets busy, and it's easy to find excuses. You may not even remember reading this book in a month or two. Like the old saying goes, it can go "in one ear and out the other." This means that you need tools to take action today. If you are the kind of person who likes to do a lot of research and loves facts, figures and statistics, then reread this book a few more times as you implement.

If you're the type of person who doesn't need too much information to make a decision, then get started today and jump right in. Essentially, you have *three options*:

One, go on your own with this information and do the best with what you have in your toolbelt right now. Use these principles and strategies to make the best of your practice and maintain the good things you already have working for you.

Two, make a few small changes with the help of your practice team members. Meet regularly and break each one down by week. After a while, you'll be able to look back and notice some significant improvements in the experience, profitability and culture in your practice.

Three, put my team to work for you, which means you can give my office a call or contact us online for a complimentary 30-minute growth consultation, to see if you are a candidate for the practice growth options we offer today.

I wish you well in your endeavors. I really enjoyed putting this book together with practice owners like you in mind. I'd love your feedback on how the book has helped you (good or bad). Please share your thoughts by leaving a review about the book on Amazon.com, Kindle or your favorite book website.

Chapter 11 Summary:

- The most important part of your practice is the experience that your patients have at every visit.

- Rethink the experience of both your new patients, existing patients, and even prospective patients. Revisit your strategy and improve this experience yearly.

- Most practice owners will not constantly improve the patient experience, which is why most practices are average.

- Get out of the office and take your team to dinner once in a while.

- Network with your community.

- Remember that relationships are far more valuable than money.

- Having the right mindset and the right methods are equal partners to your success.

- There is no easy button, but going the extra mile is what gives you the opportunity to be different.

- Do not expect perfection, but always strive for it.

- Be more than just a dentist or practice owner to your team. Be an example. Be a leader!

References

CHAPTER 1

- Diamond Story from AmericanRhetoric.com

CHAPTER 2:

- Only 11% said they'd go to Walmart: https://www.beckersdental.com/dentists/35369-walmart-health-offers-25-teeth-cleaning.html

- Dentists 1 in 3 underutilized: https://jada.ada.org/article/S0002-8177(15)00391-8/fulltext

- Workforce: https://www.ada.org/en/science-research/health-policy-institute/dental-statistics/workforce

- Dentists per 100,000 ADA: https://www.ada.org/~/media/ADA/Science%20and%20Research/HPI/Files/HPIData_SOD_2019.xlsx?la=en

- Average practice revenues in US: https://www.ada.org/en/science-research/health-policy-institute/dental-statistics/income-billing-and-other-dentistry-statistics

- Oversupply: http://www.jdentaled.org/content/81/8/eS146

- Dentists graduating in 2040: http://www.jdentaled.org/content/81/8/eS146

CHAPTER 3:

- Gold rush: Flexport.com

- $ sign invented: WSJ.com

- Trillion Dollar Stocks: Yahoo finance

- Top reasons patients seek orthodontic treatment: http://www.orthodrehab.org/article.asp?issn=2349-5243;year=2016;volume=7;issue=3;spage=89;epage=91;aulast=Jayachandar

- Top 3 reasons patients avoid the dentist study: https://www.ncbi.nlm.nih.gov/pubmed/27351733
- Top keywords searched: https://conversionsmiles.com/2018/04/29/2018-dental-keywords-list/

CHAPTER 4:

- Fair Consumer Health, Top Keyword Search 2019

CHAPTER 5:

- Apple struggles: investors.com

CHAPTER 6:

- February 2020 WSJ.com (2 separate articles)
- May 2020 Dentaltown Magazine

CHAPTER 7:

- *The Anatomy of Hope: How People Prevail In The Face Of Illness,* by Jerome Groopman, M.D., page 155
- "Why We Fail To Reach Goals: Our Brains Begin With One Focus, But Closing The Deal Requires Another" -David DiSalvo, Forbes.com, original study from Science Direct - https://www.sciencedirect.com/science/article/pii/S0166432819313889
- 2011 article, adweek.com
- The book *Traction* by Gino Wickman
- *The Book of Secrets: Unlocking the Hidden Dimensions of Your Life*, by Dr. Deepak Chopra.

CHAPTER 10

- https://www.statista.com/statistics/191043/us-consumer-spending-on-books-since-2002/
- Article by Juan Carlos Arancibia, March 2020, Investors.com

About Tyler Williams, D.D.S.

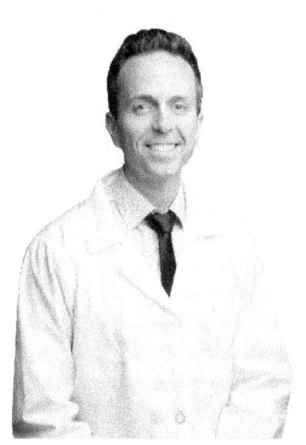

Dr. Tyler Williams is a full-time practicing dentist and the founder of Pinecrest Dental (his practice) and Pinecrest Practice Growth, a results-oriented growth program for dental practices. He is a proud husband and father of three.

He has written numerous articles for *Dentistry Today*, *The Profitable Dentist* and *Dental Economics*, the *ADA News* and the Utah Dental Association. He is the author of two other books, *Reason to Smile: 11 Keys to Your Best Oral Health Ever*, and *The Consumer's Guide to Dental Implants: 3 Keys Every Adult Needs to Know About a Smile Transformation*.

Dr. Williams has been featured on ABC's "Good Things Utah," NBC News Radio, "The One Thing" marketing podcast, Sirius XM Radio, UK Health Radio, KTALK Utah radio, and in several national dental research publications, including reviewing articles for the Academy of General Dentistry's *General Dentistry* journal. He has had several published articles in online and print journals, including: *Dental Economics, Dentistry IQ, ADA News, Dentistry Today,* and *The Profitable Dentist*. Dr. Williams has been selected as a Top Dentist in Utah by the International Association of Dentists, and spotlighted in the renowned publication, *Leading Physicians of the World*. He has also been recognized as one of America's Best Dentists for the past eight years in a row.

Dr. Williams is a member of the American Academy of Implant Dentistry, the American Academy of Facial Esthetics, the American Dental Association, and the Utah Dental Association. He has also been recognized as one of the most influential dentists in Utah by Kleer's list of Most Influential Dentists in America.

He is currently the owner of Pinecrest Practice Growth, which helps preserve independent dentistry while helping practice owners maximize the growth and opportunity within their existing practice. Dr. Williams enjoys being a speaker and instructor on dental implants with the Implant Institute. He is a real, "wet fingered dentist," and has completed thousands of dental implants and restorative procedures.

His dental practice focuses on restorative dentistry and oral-systemic health for a better quality of life.

(To contact Dr. Williams, please call (801) 512-2987, or visit yourpracticegrowth.com.)

UNLOCK MORE <u>FREE BONUSES</u>, VIDEOS, AND TOOLS INCLUDED WITH THIS BOOK, AT yourpracticegrowthbonuses.com

www.ingramcontent.com/pod-product-compliance
Lightning Source LLC
Chambersburg PA
CBHW052357220526
45465CB00003BB/1147